# Sport Psychology
# for Youth Coaches

# Sport Psychology for Youth Coaches

## Developing Champions in Sports and Life

RONALD E. SMITH
AND
FRANK L. SMOLL

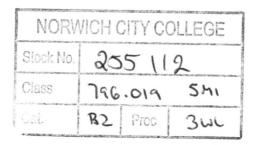
ROWMAN & LITTLEFIELD PUBLISHERS, INC.
*Lanham • Boulder • New York • Toronto • Plymouth, UK*

Published by Rowman & Littlefield Publishers, Inc.
A wholly owned subsidary of The Rowman & Littlefield Publishing Group, Inc.
4501 Forbes Boulevard, Suite 200, Lanham, Maryland 20706
www.rowman.com

10 Thornbury Road, Plymouth PL6 7PP, United Kingdom

Distributed by National Book Network

British Library Cataloguing in Publication Information Available

**Library of Congress Cataloging-in-Publication Data**

Smith, Ronald Edward, 1940–
  Sport psychology for youth coaches : developing champions in sports and life /
Ronald E. Smith and Frank L. Smoll.
    p. cm.
  Includes bibliographical references and index.
  ISBN 978-1-4422-1715-7 (pbk. : alk. paper) — ISBN 978-1-4422-1716-4
(electronic)
  1. Sports for children—Psychological aspects. 2. Coaches (Athletics) I. Smoll,
Frank L. II. Title.
  GV709.2.S535 2012
  796.019—dc23

                                                                    2012017733

♾™ The paper used in this publication meets the minimum requirements of
American National Standard for Information Sciences—Permanence of Paper for
Printed Library Materials, ANSI/NISO Z39.48-1992.

Printed in the United States of America

# Contents

**I**

# DEVELOPING A
# COACHING PHILOSOPHY

# 1

# Athletic Competition for Children and Adolescents

## Why Youth Sports?

This book is for you, the youth sport coach. We wrote it because we believe that sport participation has great potential for improving the growth and personal development of children and adolescents. Because sports are so important to youngsters, what coaches do and say can have an important long-term impact on young athletes. This book provides scientifically validated information that will help you make the sport experience constructive and enjoyable!

All coaches do as well as they can, within the limits of their awareness. The sport psychology information in these pages can increase your awareness of many of the challenges and opportunities that can arise in youth sports, and help you deal more effectively with them. The content is designed to increase the knowledge of coaches who have a strong background in sports as well as those who have relatively little athletic experience.

### THE IMPORTANCE OF PLAY

To understand the role of sports in the lives of children, we must first consider the meaning and functions of play. Animals as well as humans engage in play activities. In animals, play has long been seen as a way of learning and practicing skills and behaviors that are necessary for future survival. For example, young lions stalk and pounce on objects in their play. In children, too, play has important functions during development.

> Play is a natural training ground in
> which children learn important life skills.

From its earliest beginnings in infancy, play is a way in which children learn about the world and their place in it. Children's play serves as a training ground for developing physical abilities—skills like walking, running, and jumping that are necessary for everyday living. Play also allows children to try out and learn social behaviors and to acquire values and personality traits that will be important in adulthood. For example, they learn how to compete and cooperate with others, how to lead and follow, how to make decisions, how to assert themselves, and so on. This occurs in free-spontaneous forms of play as well as in more structured forms, such as games and sports. Thus, children's play helps them acquire physical, social, and personal skills, serving as a kind of apprenticeship for later life.

## THE GROWTH OF YOUTH SPORTS

Although children have always engaged in play, development of increasingly organized youth sport programs has occurred during the past 70 years. The growth of organized programs has been so rapid that youth sports have become a firmly established part of societies around the world.

> Youth sports are deeply rooted in social and cultural heritages.

How fast have youth sports grown? Very fast! Little League Baseball, one of the oldest programs, is a good example. It originated in 1939 in Williamsport, Pennsylvania, as a three-team league for 8- to 12-year-old boys. The program was so popular that it spread rapidly. In its 50-year anniversary season, there were some 6,800 chartered leagues in 25 countries. Little League is now comprised of a huge patchwork of nations and cultures, including Israel, Jordan, Russia, Germany, Japan, Canada, Australia, Poland, Mexico, China, Venezuela, and South Africa. Some 2.6 million 6- to 18-year-old boys and girls play Little League Baseball, including about 400,000 youngsters registered in Little League Softball.

An amazing number of youngsters participate in sports.

Programs in other sports have also shown rapid growth. Today, more opportunities to play a greater variety of sports exist than ever before, particularly for girls and young women. Estimates by the National Council of Youth Sports in 2008 indicated that about 60.3 million youngsters 6 to 18 years of age participate in agency-sponsored sports, such as Little League Baseball, the American Youth Soccer Organization, and the Boys & Girls Clubs. According to the National Federation of State High School Associations, in 2010–2011 about 7.7 million youth (4.5 million males, 3.2 million females) participated in high school sports. This situation has required the involvement of increasing numbers of adults. Accordingly, millions of men and women volunteer their time as coaches, league administrators, and officials; millions more serve as paid professionals in school-sponsored athletics. As programs have become more highly organized, parental involvement has also increased. Thus, in moving from sandlots and playgrounds to the more formalized organizations that now exist, the youth sport explosion has touched young people and adults in escalating numbers.

What factors have contributed to the rise of youth sports?

- Over the years, there has been a clear recognition of the importance of wholesome leisure-time activities for children and adolescents.
- The expansion of large cities has decreased the amount and availability of play spaces.

- Many authorities have correctly looked to sport programs as a way of reducing juvenile delinquency.
- Sport has become an increasingly central part of many cultures and personal lives. People generally have become more fitness-minded, and the mass media have brought sporting events into the homes of countless numbers of families.
- The final factor accounting for the growth of youth sports is perhaps the most important one: Sports are an enjoyable and rewarding pastime. The most essential reason for participating in sports is that they can and should provide fun and enjoyment!

Growth in the popularity and scope of youth sports and in the role that they play in the lives of children and adolescents is undeniable. But this phenomenon has generated ongoing and at times bitter debate. Serious questions have been raised about the desirability of youth sports, and answers to the questions are not simple.

## YOUTH SPORT VALUES

We have already identified some of the reasons for the rapid growth of youth sports. Obviously, the dramatic growth of youth sports could not have occurred if people didn't believe that participation is beneficial. Those who favor such programs emphasize that there are many aspects of the experience that contribute to personal development. Some supporters have pointed out that sport is a miniature life situation—one in which youngsters have to learn to cope with many of the important realities of life. Within sport, athletes learn to cooperate with others, to compete, to deal with success and failure, to develop self-control, and to take risks. Important attitudes are formed about achievement, authority, and persistence in the face of difficulty.

Adult leadership can be one of the truly positive features of organized sport programs. Knowledgeable coaches can help young athletes acquire physical skills and begin to master a sport. Higher levels of physical fitness can be promoted by such guidance. The coach can become a significant adult in an athlete's life and can have a huge positive influence on personal and social development. Likewise, the involvement of parents can bring families closer together and heighten the value of the experience for young athletes.

**Youth sports have both desirable and undesirable features.**

Youth sports have more than their share of critics. Coverage by the popular media is dominated by attacks on sport programs. Because mistreatment of children is noteworthy, sport abuses are likely to be sensationalized and widely publicized. Distortions frequently occur. One prominent sport psychologist spent 90 minutes with a newspaper reporter. For 80 minutes he discussed the positive aspects of sport programs, and for 10 minutes he talked about the problems in youth sports. The newspaper article dealt only with the problems. Furthermore, it misquoted the expert as saying that all organized sports should be eliminated for children under the age of 16. The media's overemphasis on the negative has understandably made some people question the value of youth sports.

Undoubtedly, problems can arise in sport programs, and some of these problems have been the focus of severe criticism. *Newsweek* once published a thoughtful editorial by former Major League pitcher Robin Roberts titled, "Strike Out Little League." This Hall of Fame baseball star pointed out that Little League Baseball can potentially place excessive physical and psychological strains on youngsters, and that programs sometimes exist more for the self-serving needs of the adults than for the welfare of children. Experts in child development have claimed that adult-supervised and highly organized programs can rob children of the creative benefits of spontaneous play. They suggest that children would benefit far more if adults simply left them alone to their own games and activities.

**Even the very best programs have some faults.**

Many complaints focus on the role of adults in youth sport programs. Critics have charged that some coaches are absorbed in living out their own fantasies of building sport dynasties, and that consequently they show little personal concern for their athletes. Likewise, opponents of youth sports maintain that parents sometimes live through their children's accomplishments and place tremendous pressure on them to succeed. When coaches and parents become more focused on themselves than on the quality of the children's experience, something is certainly wrong.

The negative involvement of adults in sports has been linked to such problems as the inappropriate use of drugs for training and conditioning purposes, physical injury due to excessive training and competition, and blatant cheating and dishonesty. The *Los Angeles Times* reported that one misguided coach injected oranges with amphetamines, then fed them to his 10- to 12-year-old football players to get them "up" for a game. The *Washington Post* carried a story about a mother who forged a phony birth certificate for her 17-year-old son so that he could star in a league for 14-year-olds.

Who's right? Are youth sports a symptom of a serious, widespread social disease? Or are they the salvation of our youth? The answer is neither. No reasonable person can deny that important problems do exist in some programs. Some of the criticisms are well founded and can be constructive. On the other hand, surveys have shown that the vast majority of adults and children involved in sports find them to be an enjoyable and valued part of their lives. The bottom line is that sport programs are what we make of them. They can become a source of joy and fulfillment in the life of a child, or a source of stress and disappointment.

---

A realistic appraisal of youth sports includes recognition of their positive and negative features.

---

We believe that sports have a strong positive *potential* for achieving important objectives. The question is not whether youth sports should continue to exist. They are firmly established cultural institutions. If anything, they will continue to grow in spite of the criticisms that are sometimes leveled at them. The real question is how adults can help ensure that participation in sports will be a positive experience for children and adolescents.

What can you do to help achieve the many desirable outcomes that are possible? Perhaps the key to unlocking the potential of youth sports lies in being well informed about their psychological dimensions. We hope that the sport psychology information presented in this book will assist you in your role as a successful coach.

# 2

# Sport Models and Goals

## *Kids Are Not Professionals!*

W hen children enter a sport program, they automatically assume responsibilities. But they also have rights. Adults need to respect these rights if young athletes are to have a safe and rewarding sport experience. In the United States, the National Association for Sport and Physical Education organized a Youth Sports Task Force and charged it with developing a "Bill of Rights for Young Athletes." The rights identified by these medical doctors, sport scientists, and youth sport administrators are presented in the box below.

We believe that the Bill of Rights provides a sound framework for fulfilling adult responsibilities toward young athletes. But as an important first step to guaranteeing these rights, coaches must have an understanding of the various models of sport as well as the kinds of objectives they hope to achieve. Sport models and goals are the focus of this chapter.

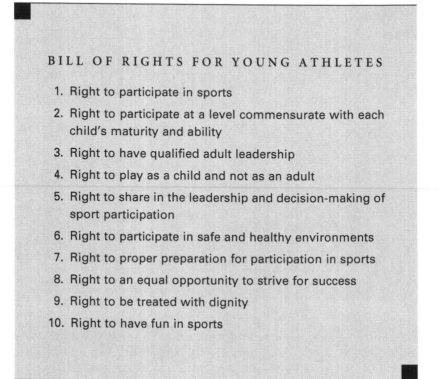

BILL OF RIGHTS FOR YOUNG ATHLETES

1. Right to participate in sports
2. Right to participate at a level commensurate with each child's maturity and ability
3. Right to have qualified adult leadership
4. Right to play as a child and not as an adult
5. Right to share in the leadership and decision-making of sport participation
6. Right to participate in safe and healthy environments
7. Right to proper preparation for participation in sports
8. Right to an equal opportunity to strive for success
9. Right to be treated with dignity
10. Right to have fun in sports

## DEVELOPMENTAL VERSUS PROFESSIONAL MODELS OF SPORT

An important issue requiring clarification is the difference between youth and professional models of sport. The major goals of professional sports are directly linked to their status in the entertainment industry. The goals of professional sports, simply stated, are to entertain, and ultimately, to make money. Financial success is of primary importance and depends heavily on a product orientation, namely, winning. Is this wrong? Certainly not! As a part of the entertainment industry, professional sports have tremendous value in all societies.

Professional sports are a huge commercial enterprise.

In the professional sport world, players are commodities to be bought, sold, and traded. Their value is based on how much they contribute to winning and profit making. They are the instruments of success on the field and at the box office, and they are dealt with as property or as cogs in a machine.

Professional athletes are often glorified by the media to create an image intended to draw paying customers and to generate interest in the team. However, many professional athletes feel that little real concern is shown for them as human beings or as contributing members of society. For example, several professional teams have reportedly turned deaf ears to reports of drug abuse by star athletes as long as the athletes continued to perform well.

---

All they seem to care about is what you did for them yesterday and what you can do for them tomorrow.

—*Willie Mays, Major League Baseball Hall of Fame player*

---

The professional coach's job is to win. Those who don't win usually join the ranks of the unemployed rather quickly and unceremoniously. No gold watches for years of service, either! A win-at-all-costs philosophy is required for advancement and, indeed, survival. Professional coaches do not receive bonuses for developing character. Their primary function is to help the franchise compete successfully for the entertainment dollar.

The developmental model of sport has a far different focus. As its name suggests, the goal is to develop the individual. The most important product is not wins or dollars but, rather, the quality of the experience for the athlete. In this sense, sport participation is an educational process whereby children and adolescents can learn to cope with realities they will face in later life. Although winning is sought after, it is by no means the primary goal. Profit is measured not in terms of dollars and cents, but rather in terms of the skills and personal characteristics that are acquired and the enjoyment of doing the activity.

> In a developmental model, sport is an arena for learning,
> where success is measured in terms of personal growth
> and development.

Sometimes, these two athletic models get confused. We are convinced that most of the problems in youth sports occur when uninformed adults erroneously impose a professional model on what should be a recreational and educational experience. This common mistake is referred to as the "professionalization" of youth sports.

## OBJECTIVES OF YOUTH SPORTS

Coaches, like young athletes, involve themselves in sports for many reasons. Youth sport objectives can range from simply providing a worthwhile leisure-time activity to laying the foundation for becoming an Olympic champion or a professional athlete. Of course, there are many other goals that may well be more appropriate. Some of them are physical, such as attaining sport skills and increasing health and fitness. Others are psychological, such as developing leadership skills, self-discipline, respect for authority, competitiveness, cooperativeness, sportsmanship, and self-confidence. These are many of the positive attributes that fall under the heading of "character."

---

The greatest contribution that sports can make to young athletes is to build character. The greatest teacher of character is on the athletic field.

—*Tom Landry, National Football League Hall of Fame coach*

---

Youth sports are also an important social activity in which youngsters can make new friends and acquaintances and become part of an ever-expanding social network. Furthermore, sports can serve to bring families closer together. Finally, of course, youth sports are (or should be) just plain *FUN!*

Fun. A term we use a lot. But what is it? Certainly it's easy to tell when people are having fun. They show it in their expression of happiness, satisfaction, and enthusiasm. Being with others, meeting challenges, feeling the drama of uncertain outcomes, becoming more skilled—all of these add to the fun of sports.

---

Fun is when I'm doing something that makes me happy just to be doing it, like playing tennis.

—*An 8-year-old girl*

---

Winning also adds to the fun, but we sell sports short if we insist that winning is the most important ingredient. In fact, several research studies reported that when children were asked where they would rather be—warming the bench on a winning team or playing regularly on a losing team—about 90 percent of them chose the losing team. The message is clear: The enjoyment of playing is more important than the satisfaction of winning.

Does your popularity as a coach depend on your won-lost record? No! In one of our own studies, we found that teams' won-lost records have nothing to do with how well young athletes liked the coaches they played for or their desire to play for the same coach again. Interestingly, however, success of the team was related to how much the children thought their parents liked the coach. The children also felt that the won-lost record influenced how much their coach liked them. It appears that, even at a very young age, children begin to tune in to the adult emphasis on winning, even though they do not yet share it themselves. What children do share is a desire to have fun.

---

It's a disgrace what we're doing in the United States and Canada. We're asking kids to compete to win. Why not ask them to compete to have fun? We're trying to build our own egos on little children.

—*Sparky Anderson, Major League Baseball Hall of Fame manager*

---

The basic right of young athletes to have fun in participating should not be neglected. One of the quickest ways to reduce fun is for adults to begin treating kids as if they were professional athletes. We need to keep in mind that young athletes are not miniature adults. They are children, and they have the right to play as children. Youth sports are, first and foremost, a play activity, and children deserve to enjoy sports in their own way. In essence, it is important that programs remain *child-centered* and do not become adult-dominated.

What are the objectives that young athletes seek to achieve? The results of two scientific surveys conducted in the United States and Canada indicated that young athletes most often say they participate in sports for the following reasons:

- To have fun
- To improve their skills and learn new skills
- To be with their friends or make new friends
- For thrills and excitement
- To succeed or win
- To become physically fit

As a concerned adult, you should ask your athletes what *they* want from sports and why *they* wish to participate. Coaches should not be guilty of forcing their own aspirations upon children and adolescents. But rather, you should make sure that young athletes have a say in determining their own destiny.

Not everyone agrees that youth sport programs succeed in achieving their goals. Critics point out that in some instances impressionable youngsters learn to swear, cheat, fight, intimidate, and hurt others. Sports provide opportunities to learn immoral values and behaviors as well as moral ones. Depending on the types of leadership provided by coaches, the experiences can result in sinners as well as saints. In the final analysis, it is not the sport itself that automatically determines the worth of the activity for the child, but rather the nature of the experiences within the program.

> All children should have an opportunity to participate
> in sports regardless of gender, race, or ability level.

Not every child may choose to participate in sports, but every child has the right to choose to participate. This includes the right to participate *fully*. Although all children cannot play every minute of every athletic event, they should have an opportunity to play a reasonable amount in all sport events. Well-informed and qualified coaches appropriately adopt the attitude that it is important to play every child for the child's sake.

Whatever your objectives may be, it is important that you become aware of them. And you must realize that none of these objectives can be achieved automatically as a result of mere participation in sports. Simply placing a youngster in a sport situation does not guarantee a positive outcome. The nature and quality of the program, which are directly dependent on your input, are prime factors in determining benefits.

**KEEPING SPORTS IN PERSPECTIVE**

Earlier in this chapter we indicated that athletics can contribute to the personal, social, and physical well-being of youngsters. Sport is an important area in the lives of many children. And for a small number, youth sports are the first phase of a journey that ends in a career in professional athletics.

I am worried about my son. He seems to have gotten things out of perspective as far as sports are concerned. Although he's only 13 years old, he is convinced that his future lies in college and professional sports. Nothing else seems to matter.

—*A young athlete's father*

To strive for high standards of athletic excellence is commendable. But coaches, parents, and athletes alike must realize that the chances of actually becoming a professional are remote. Even if a youngster appears to be a gifted athlete, the odds are overwhelming. Statistically speaking, the chances of a high school athlete becoming a professional in any sport are 1 in 12,000.

> The stiff odds against a child's becoming a college or professional athlete indicate that youth sports should not be treated as a feeder system. Instead, the focus should be on personal growth and development.

Given the reality of the situation, a career in professional sports or even participation at the college level is an unrealistic goal for the majority of young athletes. It is therefore important to impress on youngsters that sport is but one part of life for a well-rounded person. It is all too easy for young athletes to harbor fantasies of turning pro and to sacrifice other areas of their development in pursuit of that fabled status and its rewards of fame, money, and glory. As valuable as athletics can be for developing children, social and academic development, spiritual enrichment, and quality of family life should not suffer. Sports can offer both fun and fulfillment, but there is more to life than sports.

Perhaps the best advice we can give is to encourage children to participate in sports if they wish. But at the same time coaches should help athletes understand that sport participation is not an end in itself, but a means of achieving various goals. You can teach them to enjoy the process of competition for itself, rather than to focus on such end products as victories and trophies. Neither victory nor defeat should be blown out of proportion, and no coach should permit a child to define his or her self-worth purely on the basis of sport performance. By keeping sports in perspective, you can make them a source of personal growth and enrichment.

# BECOMING A BETTER COACH

# 3

# Coaching Roles and Relationships

## Influencing Young Athletes' Lives

As a coach, you probably know sport techniques and strategies, but are you prepared to deal with young athletes who rely on you to provide a worthwhile and enjoyable experience? Each youngster differs in ability and personality and has different reasons for playing a sport. Some hope to be future champions; most simply want to have fun; and others are there because their parents or friends have pressured them into participating. There are even those who wonder what they are doing there. And there you are, trying to meet the needs and expectations of a highly varied group of young personalities. As one experienced coach recalls: You are a teacher, amateur psychologist, substitute parent, and important role model—in other words, you are a coach!

### ORIENTATION TO THE PSYCHOLOGY OF COACHING

In your role as a coach, you are trying to influence the behavior of athletes in desirable ways—athletically, psychologically, and socially. That's where psychology, the science of mind and behavior, comes in. Simply stated, the psychology of coaching is nothing more than a set of principles that guide your behavior as a coach. Coaches can have different goals and different approaches to what they do, and these approaches can have very different effects on their athletes.

> A coach can be completely unaware of the influence that
> he or she is having in the life of a young athlete.

Many coaches tend to underestimate the influence they can have on the youngsters who play for them. In addition to the central role that you occupy in athletics, it is important to recognize that your influence also extends into other areas of your athletes' lives. Your actions and the attitudes and values you express help shape their view of the world and of themselves. For some young athletes, you may be a more important influence than their parents during a formative period of their lives. In some cases, the youngster may even look to you as a substitute for a parent who is missing in either a physical or a psychological sense.

Should this potential impact on a child's life scare you? Not if you have a genuine concern for youngsters and if you have established for yourself what it is you are attempting to accomplish through coaching. As a coach, you can make an important contribution that, coupled with the contributions of other responsible adults, helps a child on his or her way to a happy, productive, and well-adjusted life.

## ACHIEVEMENT IN SPORTS AND LIFE

The sport environment is a developmentally significant one, partly because it is an achievement setting of great relevance to the participants. For example, research has shown that children's motivation and investment are greater in sport activities than in classroom activities and interactions with their friends. Therefore, important lessons about achievement and the meaning of success and failure can be learned in athletics.

When conducted properly, youth sports can help youngsters acquire the kinds of attitudes, values, and skills that promote achievement and success in all areas of life. When mismanaged, sports can create fear of failure, reduce enjoyment, undermine self-worth, and counter values of fair play. Which of these consequences occurs depends largely on the type of *motivational climate* that is created by coaches. The motivational climate is critically important because it communicates different notions about what success is and what is required to be a "success."

Researchers who study achievement motivation have identified two different ways of defining success. An *ego goal orientation* is found in people who define success as winning or being better than others. They are always comparing themselves with others and don't feel successful unless they see themselves as performing better than others. Anything short of victory is failure and indicates to them that they are inferior. Carried to an extreme, the view is that "If I'm not the best, I'm the worst." For such people, the stakes are high for winning or losing, and some develop high fear of failure because, to them, failure means inferiority.

---

If you make winning games a life or death proposition, you're going to have problems. For one thing, you'll be dead a lot.

—*Dean Smith, Basketball Hall of Fame coach*

---

A second and healthier view of success is called a *mastery goal orientation*. Mastery-oriented people focus on their own effort and accomplishments instead of comparing themselves with others. In a sense, they compare themselves with themselves. They can feel success and satisfaction when they have learned something new, seen skill improvement in themselves, or given maximum effort. Even if they see themselves as less skillful than someone else, mastery-oriented people can feel competent and successful if they view themselves as doing their best to become the best they can be. In the long run, by focusing on becoming *their* best, mastery-oriented people are more likely to realize their potential and to be free of the performance-destroying fear of failure that causes some athletes to "choke" under pressure.

Success is peace of mind which is a direct result of self-satisfaction in knowing you made the effort to do the best of which you are capable.

—*John Wooden, Basketball Hall of Fame player and coach*

Coach John Wooden's perspective on success may be the most important reason why he deserves the title "Wizard of Westwood." He realized that everyone can be a success, because success relates to the effort that one puts into realizing one's personal potential.

Ego and mastery goal orientations do not develop in a vacuum; they are acquired and reinforced by significant adults. Adults create the *motivational climate* by the values they communicate (particularly about what success is) and by the behaviors they reward or punish. In youth sports, athletes' attitudes toward success and achievement develop within the motivational climate created by coaches. In an *ego-based climate*, the emphasis is on winning out over others, including both opponents and one's own teammates. It's fair to say that the following statement typifies an ego environment:

In this game, you're either a winner or a loser. Success means winning championships. Anything else is failure.

—*George Allen, Pro Football Hall of Fame coach*

In an ego-based climate, coaches often focus their attention on the most talented athletes, who have the greatest influence on winning. Effort and improvement are not emphasized as much as performance level. Coaches may encourage rivalry among teammates by comparing them openly with one another. Coaches may punish inadequate performance or mistakes with belittlement and criticism, teaching children that mistakes are to be avoided at all costs and thereby building fear of failure. Another unfortunate outcome associated with an ego climate is the willingness to win at all costs, even if rule breaking is required to gain the needed advantage. Obviously, this doesn't sound like a fun environment. And, in fact, athletes in such sport environments report much lower enjoyment than those in mastery environments.

In a *mastery-based climate*, the goal is to foster positive growth as an athlete and as a person. The emphasis is on effort, learning, and personal improvement—doing what it takes to be *your* best. To be sure, winning is valued, but in a mastery climate, the adults realize that winning takes care of itself if athletes are having fun, improving their skills, giving maximum effort, and working together, and if they are not shackled with fear of failing. Mastery climates foster an atmosphere of mutual support and encouragement, and everyone, regardless of ability, is made to feel an important part of the team.

## MASTERY CLIMATE RESEARCH RESULTS

Which type of motivational climate is best for youth sports? Scientific research has provided a clear answer, and it is the same answer that has been shown in school and work settings. Mastery climates consistently have more positive effects on both achievement and on psychological factors. Seven of the beneficial effects are summarized here.

1. In mastery climates, young athletes are more likely to develop intrinsic (internal) motivation for the activity, enjoying the activity for itself. In ego climates, participation is not enjoyed for itself but instead is a means toward some other, extrinsic (external) end, such as social status and recognition.

2. Mastery climates are associated with greater sport enjoyment. In ego climates, pressures to outperform others decrease enjoyment if you're not "top dog." Not surprisingly, more kids drop out of sports from ego climates because competitive pressures decrease fun.

3. Mastery climates minimize fear of failure, because of the emphasis on effort, persistence, and improvement, all of which are within the athlete's control. Ego climates foster fear of failure because comparisons with others (whose performance one can't control) and concerns about ability increase anxiety.

4. Mastery climates tend to increase self-esteem because children are rewarded and take pride in their own improvement and effort. In ego climates, athletes may not feel good about themselves unless they outperform others, and a failure to do so may diminish feelings of self-worth.

5. In mastery climates, athletes come to believe that effort is the key to success, and they value hard work and cooperation with others. In other words, they internalize John Wooden's definition of success, striving to become the best they can be. In ego climates, athletes believe that ability and "getting an edge" over others is what governs success. They are therefore more willing to cheat or use intimidation to win.

6. Mastery climates, whether in sports or in school, promote faster and better skill development and higher performance than do ego climates. When athletes are enjoying themselves, focusing on effort and improvement, and are not hampered by fear of failing, winning takes care of itself. In such cases, coaches find that their teams are actually more successful.

7. In terms of athletes' ratings of how much fun they had and how much they liked playing for their coach, one study showed that a mastery climate was about 10 times more influential than was the teams' won-lost records.

Given these consistent research results, it is no accident that the guidelines found in this book are designed to help coaches create a mastery-based motivational climate. Further, the findings on performance show that coaches do not need to choose between winning and providing a mastery climate. Both goals can be achieved at the same time. Athletes are likely to learn skills faster and ultimately perform better if they are having fun in a supportive environment that focuses on effort and improvement, and in which mistakes are viewed as ways of learning rather than things to be feared.

Buying into a mastery orientation means that winning becomes something different than collecting "Ws" and league championships. Let's examine this conception of what it means to be a "winner."

## A HEALTHY PHILOSOPHY OF WINNING

In terms of the educational benefits of sport, young athletes can learn from both winning and losing. But for this to occur, winning must be put in a *healthy* perspective. We have therefore developed a four-part philosophy of winning designed to maximize athletes' enjoyment of sport and their chances of receiving the positive outcomes of participation.

1. *Winning isn't everything, nor is it the only thing.* Young athletes can't possibly learn from winning and losing if they think the only objective is to beat their opponents. Does this mean that you should not try to build winning teams? Definitely not! As a form of competition, sport involves a contest between opposing individuals or teams. It would be naive and unrealistic to believe that winning is not an important goal in sports. But it is not the most important objective.

Youngsters should leave your program having enjoyed relating to you and their teammates, feeling better about themselves, having improved their skills, and looking forward to future sport participation. When this happens, something far more valuable has been accomplished than having a winning record or winning a league championship.

2. *Failure is not the same thing as losing.* Athletes should not view losing as a sign of failure or as a threat to their personal value. They should be taught that losing a competition is not a reflection of their own self-worth. In other words, when individuals or teams lose, it does not mean that they are worth less than if they had won. In fact, some valuable lessons can be learned from losing. Children can learn to persist in the face of obstacles and to support each other even when they do not achieve victory.

3. *Success does not depend on winning.* Thus, neither success nor failure need depend on the outcome of a competition or on a won-lost record. Winning and losing apply to the outcome of a competition, whereas success and failure do not. How, then, can we define success in sports?

4. *Athletes should be taught that success is found in striving for victory.* The important idea is that *success is related to effort*! Effort is within

athletes' zone of control. They have only limited control over the outcome that is achieved. If you can impress on your athletes that they are never "losers" if they give maximum effort, you are giving them a priceless gift that will assist them in many of life's tasks. A youth soccer coach had the right idea when he told his team, "You kids are always winners when you try your best! But sometimes the other team will score more goals."

---

I have no control over results. All I can do is play to the best of my abilities. Success is me giving everything that I have.

—*Ichiro Suzuki, Major League Baseball star*

---

How can you teach an effort-oriented philosophy of winning? First, have regular discussions about it. You must continually remind athletes about the importance of effort. Second, back up your words with actions. In other words, don't just talk about effort, do something about it! Many of the guidelines presented in the next chapter are specifically designed to teach athletes the value of effort. Third, help athletes set individualized goals specific to them, and encourage them to work toward them. If they're working on a technical skill, try to find a way to measure their performance so they can see their improvement. Use praise and recognition to reward effort and improvement. Encourage effort and persistence, telling athletes that skills develop gradually, not all at once. In a mastery climate, the "most improved player" award is just as important as the "most valuable player." Finally, convey to your athletes that mistakes are one of the best ways to learn, and that they needn't fear making them. John Wooden referred to mistakes as "stepping stones to achievement" because they provide the feedback needed to improve performance.

# 4

# The Mastery Approach to Coaching

## *Applying Sport Psychology*

There are two basic approaches to influencing people, both of which are used by coaches. The *positive approach* is designed to increase desirable behaviors by motivating athletes to perform them and by rewarding (reinforcing) the athletes when they do. This "relationship style" goes hand-in-hand with the healthy philosophy of winning presented earlier. And it creates a mastery-based climate, so we will refer to it as the *Mastery Approach to Coaching*, or the Mastery Approach, throughout the remainder of the book.

The *negative approach*, which is often present in an ego-based climate, involves attempts to eliminate athletes' mistakes through the use of punishment and criticism. The motivating factor in this "command style" is fear. Punitive coaching behaviors have many undesirable side effects that can actually interfere with what a coach is trying to accomplish. Using a negative approach is the fastest way to instill fear of failure and to create resentment and hostility.

Both coaching styles are used at all levels of competition. However, the effectiveness of the Mastery Approach has been scientifically validated. This means that we are not shooting from the hip with personal beliefs or so-called armchair psychology about what we think will work. Rather, the behavioral guidelines (leadership principles) comprising the Mastery Approach were derived from our research on how coaching behaviors actually affect young athletes. The guidelines were also evaluated in numerous studies conducted in real-life sport settings. In these studies, groups of coaches were randomly placed in either (a) an experimental (training) condition in which they learned the guidelines, or (b) a control condition in which training did not occur. Athletes' attitudes and psychological characteristics were measured at the beginning and end of the season so that the effects of the training and control conditions could be compared. The results consistently confirmed that the *Mastery Approach to Coaching* produces the following outcomes:

- Fosters positive coach-athlete relations and greater mutual respect
- Increases the amount of fun that athletes experience
- Creates greater team cohesion and a more supportive athletic setting
- Promotes higher mastery-oriented achievement goals in sports and in school
- Increases athletes' self-esteem
- Reduces performance-destroying anxiety and fear of failure
- Decreases athlete dropout rates from approximately 30 percent to 5 percent
- Produces equally positive effects on boys' and girls' teams

It's not surprising that prominent coaches recognize and practice the power of the Mastery Approach.

---

I try never to plant a negative seed. I try to make every comment a positive comment. There's a lot of scientific evidence to support positive management.

—*Jimmy Johnson, former National Football League coach*

---

There are three important points to emphasize about the leadership principles that comprise the Mastery Approach. First, they are *not sport specific*, which means they can be applied in all sports. Second, they are *not age specific*, so they can be used across all levels of competition. Third, they are *not restricted to use in sports*. For example, because parenting is a form of leadership, you can use these principles in raising your children.

You likely will recognize that many of the recommended coaching behaviors are things you already do. However, the challenge is to integrate *new* procedures into your personal coaching style. This will require dedication and effort on your part. We now present the Mastery Approach behavioral guidelines.

## REACTIVE COACHING BEHAVIORS

Reactive coaching behaviors occur immediately after individual athlete or team behaviors. They include responses to (a) desirable performance and effort, (b) mistakes, (c) misbehaviors by athletes, and (d) violations of team rules.

### Reacting to Good Plays and Effort: The "Reinforcement Power" of Coaches

Our concern with influencing athletes' behavior in a desirable way involves the process of learning. It is well known that people tend to repeat behaviors that produce pleasant outcomes. In this context, reinforcement refers to any event occurring after a behavior that increases the likelihood that the behavior will occur again in the future. (It is similar to the more familiar concept of reward, but psychologists prefer the term *reinforcement* because what is "rewarding" for one person may not be a reward for another.) The cornerstone of the *Mastery Approach to Coaching* is the skilled use of reinforcement to increase athletic motivation and to strengthen desired behaviors.

> The most effective way to build desirable behaviors
> is to use your "reinforcement power."

Choosing a reinforcer is not usually difficult. But in some cases, your creativity and sensitivity to the needs of individual athletes might be tested. Potential reinforcers include social behaviors such as verbal praise, nonverbal signs such as smiles or applause, and acceptable forms of physical contact such as a high five or a fist bump. They also include the opportunity to engage in certain activities (such as extra batting practice) or to play with a particular piece of equipment.

Social reinforcers are most frequently employed in athletics. But even here you must decide what is most likely to be effective with each athlete. One athlete might find praise given in the presence of others highly reinforcing, whereas another might find it embarrassing.

> The best way to find an effective reinforcer is
> to get to know each athlete's likes and dislikes.

In some instances you may elect to praise an entire unit or group of athletes. At other times, reinforcement may be directed at one athlete. If at all possible, it is a good idea to use a variety of reinforcers and vary what you say and do so that you do not begin to sound like a broken record. In the final analysis, the acid test of your choice of reinforcer is whether it affects behavior in the desired manner.

Here are some principles for the effective use of your reinforcement power.

1. *Be liberal with reinforcement.* In our research, the single most important difference between coaches to whom athletes responded most favorably and those they evaluated least favorably was the frequency with which coaches reinforced desirable behaviors. You can increase the effectiveness of verbal reinforcement by combining it with a specific description of the desirable behavior that the athlete just performed. For example, you might say, "Way to go, Chris! You kept your head in there on the follow-through." In this way, you combine the power of the reinforcement with an instructional reminder of what the athlete should do. It also cues the athlete about what to concentrate on.

Reinforcement should not be restricted to the learning and performance of sport skills. Rather, it should also be liberally applied to strengthen desirable psychosocial behaviors (e.g., teamwork, leadership, sportsmanship). Look for positive things, reinforce them, and you will see them increase. Reinforce the little things that others might not notice. We are not promoting a sickeningly sweet approach with which there is a danger of looking phony and losing credibility. When sincerely given, reinforcement does not spoil youngsters; it gives them something to strive for. Remember, whether athletes show it or not, the reinforcement you give them helps strengthen the good feelings they have about themselves.

2. *Have realistic expectations and consistently reinforce achievement.* Gear your expectations to individual ability levels. For some athletes, merely running up and down the field or court without tripping is a significant accomplishment worthy of praise. For those who are more skilled, set your expectations at appropriately higher levels.

Successful coaching requires skillful use of reinforcement.

In many instances, complex skills can be broken down into their component subskills. You can then concentrate on one subskill at a time until it is mastered. For example, a football coach might choose to concentrate entirely on the pattern run by a pass receiver with no concern about whether or not the pass is completed. This is where your knowledge of the sport and of the mastery levels of your individual athletes is crucial. If you are attentive to their instructional needs and progress, athletes can enjoy lots of support and reinforcement long before they have completely mastered the entire skill.

Start with what the athlete is currently capable of doing and then gradually require more and more of the athlete before reinforcement is given. It is important that the shift in demands be realistic and that the steps be small enough that the athlete can master them and be reinforced. Used correctly, progressive reinforcement is one of the most powerful of all the positive control techniques.

Once skills are well learned, gradually shift your reinforcement to a partial schedule. This means that some correct responses are reinforced, and some are not. Research has shown that behaviors reinforced on partial schedules persist much longer in the absence of reinforcement than do actions that have been reinforced only on a continuous schedule. As casino owners are well aware, people will put a great many coins into slot machines, which operate on partial schedules. In contrast, they are unlikely to persist long in putting coins into soft drink machines that do not deliver. Thus, the key is to start with continuous reinforcement until the skill is mastered. Then shift gradually to partial reinforcement to maintain a high level of motivation and performance.

3. *Give reinforcement for desirable behavior as soon as it occurs.* The timing of reinforcement is another important consideration. Other things being equal, the sooner reinforcement occurs after a response, the stronger are its effects. Thus, whenever possible, try to reinforce a desired behavior as soon as it occurs. If this is not possible, however, try to find an opportunity to praise the athlete later on.

4. *Reinforce effort as much as results.* This guideline has direct relevance to developing a healthy philosophy of winning. To put this philosophy into practice, tell your athletes that their efforts are valued and appreciated, and back up your words with action (i.e., reinforcement). Athletes' efforts should not be ignored.

---

**Don't take athletes' effort for granted.**

---

As a coach, you have a right to demand total effort. And this is perhaps the most important thing of all for you to reinforce. We stated earlier (chapter 3) that athletes have complete control over how much effort they make, but they have only limited control over the outcome of their efforts. By looking for and reinforcing athletes' efforts, you can encourage them to continue or increase their output.

### Reacting to Mistakes

Many athletes are motivated to achieve because of a positive desire to succeed. They appear to welcome and peak under pressure. Unfortunately, many others are motivated primarily by fear of failure, and consequently they dread critical situations and the possibility of failure and disapproval. Fear of failure is an athlete's worst enemy. It can harm performance, and it reduces the enjoyment of competing. The way you react to athletes' mistakes plays a major role in either creating or combating fear of failure.

> If you manage things right, mistakes can be golden opportunities to improve performance.

A typical attitude about mistakes is that they are totally bad and must be avoided at all costs. Rather than focusing on the negative aspects of mistakes, recognize that they are not only unavoidable, but that they have a positive side as well. As noted earlier, John Wooden referred to mistakes as the "stepping stones to achievement." They provide information that is needed to improve performance. By communicating this concept to athletes in word and action, you can help them accept and learn from their mistakes.

In addition, remember that what you say and do has an important effect on athletes. Thus, deal honestly and openly with your own mistakes. When you have the confidence and courage to admit that you made a mistake, you provide a valuable role model. Such a model is important for developing a sense of tolerance for human error and for reducing fear of failure. Remember, the positive approach is designed to create a positive motive to achieve rather than a fear of failure.

You must know quite well that you are not perfect, that you're going to make mistakes. But you must not be afraid of making mistakes or you won't do anything, and that's the greatest mistake of all. We must have initiative and act and know that we're going to fail at times, for failure will only make us stronger if we accept it properly.

—*John Wooden, Basketball Hall of Fame player and coach*

1. *Give encouragement immediately after a mistake.* Athletes know when they make a poor play and often feel embarrassed about it. This is the time they are in most need of your encouragement and support.

2. *If an athlete knows how to correct the mistake, encouragement alone is sufficient.* Telling an athlete what he or she already knows may be more irritating than helpful. Do not overload athletes with unnecessary input. If you are not sure if the athlete knows how to correct the mistake, ask the athlete for confirmation.

3. *When appropriate, give corrective instruction after a mistake, but always do so in an encouraging and positive way.* In line with the Mastery Approach, mistakes can be excellent opportunities to provide technical instruction. There are three keys to giving such instruction:

- Know *what* to do—the technical aspects of correcting performance.
- Know *how* to do it—the teaching-learning approach.
- Know *when* to do it—timing.

Most athletes respond best to immediate correction, and instruction is particularly meaningful at that time. However, some athletes respond much better to instruction if you wait for some time after the mistake. Because of individual differences, such athletes are more receptive to your instruction when it is given later.

> In giving corrective instruction, don't focus on the mistake but emphasize the good things that will happen if the athlete follows your instruction.

When you are correcting mistakes, a three-part teaching approach is recommended. In the following example, a football player has dropped a pass because he took his eyes off the ball:

- Start with a *compliment*; find something the athlete did correctly ("Way to hustle. You really ran a good pattern!"). This is intended to reinforce a desirable behavior and create an open attitude on the part of the athlete.

- Give the *future-oriented instruction* ("If you follow the ball all the way into your hands, you'll catch those just like a pro does."). Emphasize the desired *future* outcome rather than the negative one that just occurred.

- End with another *positive statement* ("Hang in there. You're going to get even better if you work at it."). This "positive sandwich" approach (two positive communications wrapped around the instruction) is designed to make the athlete positively self-motivated to perform correctly rather than negatively motivated to avoid failure and disapproval.

4. *Don't punish when things go wrong.* Punishment is any consequence that decreases the future occurrence of a behavior. Punishment can be administered in either of two forms: (a) by doing something aversive, such as painful physical contact or verbal abuse, and (b) by taking something that is valued away from the athlete, or more technically, by removing positive reinforcers that are usually available to an individual, such as privileges, social interactions, or possessions. With respect to the first form, punishment is not just yelling at athletes. It can be any form of disapproval, tone of voice, or action. Constant use of such punishment leads to resentment of the coach and is a probable factor contributing to lack of enjoyment and athletic dropout.

5. *Don't give corrective instruction in a hostile or punitive way.* Although a coach may have good intentions in giving instruction, this kind of negative communication is more likely to increase frustration and create resentment than to improve performance.

Does this mean that you should avoid all criticism and punishment? Certainly not! Sometimes these behaviors are necessary for instructional or disciplinary purposes. But they should be used sparingly. If you feel that you must use punishment, do it only as a last resort, and do it in such a way that it's clear that you dislike the *behavior,* not the person. The negative approach should *never* be the primary approach to athletes.

Although abusive coaches may enjoy success and may even be admired by some of their athletes, they run the risk of losing other athletes who could contribute to the team's success and who could profit personally from an athletic experience. Coaches who succeed through the use of punishment and intimidation usually do so because (a) they are also able to communicate caring for their athletes as people, so that the abuse is not taken personally; (b) they have very talented athletes; and/ or (c) they are such skilled teachers and strategists that these abilities override their negative behaviors. In other words, such coaches win *in spite of*, not because of, the negative approach.

### Misbehaviors, Lack of Attention—Maintaining Order and Discipline

Problems of athlete misbehavior during practices and competitions (games, matches, meets) can indeed become serious. In dealing effectively with this, recognize that youngsters want clearly defined limits and structure. They do not like unpredictability and inconsistency. On the other hand, they do not like it when you play the role of a policeman or enforcer. Thus, the objective is to structure the situation so that you can teach discipline without having to constantly read the riot act to keep things under control. The statements below are guidelines to maintaining order and discipline.

1. *Maintain order by establishing clear expectations and a "team rule" concept.*

2. *Involve athletes in forming behavioral guidelines and work to build team unity in achieving them.*

3. *Strive to achieve a balance between freedom and structure.*

These guidelines promote a cooperative approach to leadership in that athletes are given a share of the responsibility for determining their own governance. The rationale for this approach is that people are more willing to live by rules (a) when they have a hand in setting them, and

(b) when they have made a public commitment to follow them. There is considerable research support for this rationale in psychology.

Team rules should be developed early in the season. In helping athletes share responsibility for forming rules, use the following four-part procedures.

- Explain why team rules are necessary: "Rules and regulations are an important part of the game. If we have team rules, they will keep things organized and efficient. This will increase our chances of achieving individual and team goals."
- Explain why the team rules should be something that they can agree on as a group: "The rules will be *your* rules, and it will be *your* responsibility to follow them."
- Solicit suggestions and ideas, and listen to what athletes say to show that their ideas and feelings are valued: "What rules do you want to have?"
- Incorporate athletes' input into a reasonable set of rules. Rules should provide structure and yet not be too rigid. The following are examples of such rules: (a) Be prepared and focused during practice and competition. (b) Give maximum effort at all times. (c) Treat others like you want to be treated.

In addition to formulating a set of team rules, be sure to discuss the kinds of penalties that you will use for breaking them. Here again, athletes should participate in determining the consequences that will follow rule violations. And of course, your role includes ensuring that the consequences are realistic.

> Teaching self-discipline is an important youth sport objective.

The advantage of this approach is that it places the responsibility where it belongs—on the athletes themselves. In this way, team discipline can help develop self-discipline. Then, when someone breaks a team rule, it is not the individual versus *your* rules, but the breaking of *their own rules.*

4. *Emphasize that during competition, all members of the team are part of it, even those on the bench.* This rule can play an important role in building team cohesion and mutual support among teammates.

5. *Use reinforcement to strengthen team participation, discipline, and unity.* By strengthening desirable behaviors, you can help prevent misbehaviors from occurring. In other words, you can prevent misbehaviors by using the positive approach to strengthen their opposites. Similarly, instances of teamwork and of athletes' support and encouragement of each other should be acknowledged and reinforced whenever possible. This not only strengthens these desirable behaviors but also creates an atmosphere in which you yourself are serving as a positive model by supporting them.

> Taking the time to develop team rules
> is easier than dealing with violations.

### Dealing with Team Rule Violations

When you have team rules, you can expect that they will be broken from time to time. As youngsters establish independence and personal identity, part of the process involves testing the limits imposed by adult authority figures—people like you! Because this is a very natural process in development, you should not feel persecuted or take it too personally. It happens with all youth coaches (as well as high school, college, and professional coaches) from time to time, and therefore these recommendations for dealing with team rules are presented.

1. *Allow the athlete to explain his or her actions.* There may be a reasonable cause for what the athlete did or did not do, and lines of communication should be kept open.

2. *Be consistent and impartial.* In other words, avoid showing favoritism. Treat *all* athletes—the stars and the subs—equally and fairly. Fairness builds respect.

3. *Don't express anger and a punitive attitude.* And of course, never take action for the purpose of retaliating.

4. *Don't lecture or embarrass the athlete.* It simply is not necessary or beneficial.

5. *Focus on the fact that a team policy has been broken, placing the responsibility on the athlete.* This should be done without degrading the individual or making the athlete feel he or she is in your doghouse. Remind the athlete that a rule was violated that he or she agreed to follow, and because of that a penalty must be paid. This focuses the responsibility where it belongs—on the athlete—and helps build a sense of personal accountability.

> A penalty must be paid for violating a rule
> that the team, not the coach, established.

6. *When giving penalties, it is best to deprive athletes of something they value.* For example, participation can be temporarily suspended by having the player sit off to the side ("time out" or "penalty box"). Taking away playing time or a starting position are also effective penalties.

7. *Don't use physical measures that could become aversive by being used to punish (e.g., running laps, doing push-ups).* It is not educationally sound to have beneficial physical activities become unpleasant because they have been used as punishment.

## SPONTANEOUS/SELF-INITIATED COACHING BEHAVIORS

### Getting Positive Things to Happen

1. *Set a good example of behavior.* Children learn a great deal by watching and imitating others. Imitation (or modeling) is an important

form of learning for children. Most athletes will have a high regard for you, and consequently they are likely to copy your behaviors and deal with sport situations in similar ways. Athletes probably learn as much from what you do as from what you say! Because of this, it is important that you portray a role model worthy of respect from athletes, officials, parents, and other coaches as well.

---

A careful man I want to be,
A little fellow follows me.
I do not dare to go astray,
For fear he'll go the selfsame way.

—*Rev. Claude Wisdom White, Sr., author/poet*

---

2. *Encourage effort, don't demand results.* This is another Mastery Approach guideline that applies to the healthy philosophy of winning presented in chapter 3. Most young athletes are already motivated to develop their skills and play well. By appropriate use of encouragement, you can help increase their natural enthusiasm. If, however, youngsters are encouraged to strive for unrealistic standards of achievement, they may feel like failures when they do not reach their goals. Therefore, it is important to base your encouragement on reasonable expectations. Again, emphasizing effort rather than outcome can help avoid problems. This concept is illustrated in the words of John Wooden:

---

You cannot find a player who ever played for me at UCLA that can tell you that he ever heard me mention "winning" a basketball game. He might say I inferred a little here and there, but I never mentioned winning. Yet the last thing that I told my players, just prior to tip-off, before we would go on the floor was, "When the game is over, I want your head up—and I know of only one way for your head to be up— and that's for you to know that you did your best. . . . This means to do the best you can do. That's the best; no one can do more. . . . You made that effort."

---

3. *In giving encouragement, be selective so that it is meaningful.* In other words, be supportive without acting like a cheerleader.

4. *Never give encouragement or instruction in a sarcastic or degrading manner.* For example, "Come on gang, we're only down 37-1. Let's really come back and make it 37-2!" Even if you do not intend the sarcasm to be harmful, youngsters sometimes do not understand the meaning of this type of communication. They may think that you are amusing others at their expense, resulting in irritation or frustration or both.

> The *Mastery Approach to Coaching* is characterized by liberal use of reinforcement and encouragement.

5. *Encourage athletes to be supportive of each other, and reinforce them when they are.* Encouragement can become contagious and contribute to building team cohesion. Communicate the enthusiasm you feel, which then carries over to your athletes. The best way to do this is by (a) presenting an enthusiastic coaching model, and (b) reinforcing athlete behaviors that promote team unity.

**Creating a Good Learning Atmosphere**

Young athletes expect you to help them satisfy their desire to become as skilled as possible. Therefore, you must establish your teaching role as early as possible. In doing this, emphasize the fun and learning part of sport, and let your athletes know that a primary coaching goal is to help them develop their athletic potential.

There is nothing mysterious about developing a good team, because coaching is nothing more than teaching. Coaches impart the techniques to the players. The better job they do, the better job the players will do.

—*John McKay, former University of Southern California and professional football coach*

During each practice or competition, be sure that every youngster gets recognized at least once. Athletes who usually get the most recognition are (a) stars, or (b) those who are causing problems. Average athletes need attention too! A good technique is to occasionally keep a count of how often you talk with each athlete to make sure that your personal contact is being appropriately distributed.

1. *Always give instructions positively.* Emphasize the good things that will happen if athletes do it right rather than focusing totally on the negative things that will occur if they don't. As stated earlier, this approach motivates athletes to make desirable things happen rather than building fear of making mistakes.

2. *When giving instructions, be clear and concise.* Young athletes have a short attention span. In addition, they may not be able to understand the technical aspects of performance in great detail. Therefore, provide simple yet accurate teaching cues, using as little verbal explanation as possible.

3. *Show athletes the correct technique.* Demonstrate or model skills being taught. If you cannot perform the skill correctly, use accomplished athletes for demonstration purposes. A proper teaching sequence includes the following:

- Introduce a skill with a demonstration.
- Provide an accurate but brief verbal explanation.
- Have athletes actively practice the skill.

Because of the way in which children respond to teaching efforts, a Chinese proverb applies: "I hear and I forget. I see and I remember. I do and I understand."

4. *Be patient and don't expect or demand more than maximum effort.* Acquisition of sport skills does not occur overnight. The gradual learning process is characterized by periods of improvement alternating with times in which no progress occurs regardless of the effort expended. Not only must you be persistent, but athletes must be convinced to stick to it and continue to give their best effort.

When an athlete has had a poor practice or a rough competition, the youngster should not go home feeling bad. He or she should get some kind of support from you—a pat on the back, a kind word ("Hey, we're going to work that out. I know what you're going through, but everyone has days like that sometimes."). Athletes should not leave feeling detached from you or feeling like a "loser."

5. *Reinforce effort and progress.* Again, the foundation of the Mastery Approach is the administration of reinforcement for effort as well as desirable motor performance and psychosocial behavior.

## GAINING ATHLETES' RESPECT

All of what we have emphasized up to now is relevant to gaining the respect of your athletes. There are two keys to gaining such respect:

- Show your athletes that you can teach them to develop their skills and that you are willing to make the effort to do so.
- Be a fair and considerate leader. Show them that you care about them as individuals and that you are glad to be coaching them.

---

Treat athletes like they are your family. Your program discipline breeds self-discipline. Love: Find something in each player to love them for. Don't spoil them—no special deals or star treatment.

—*Don James, College Football Hall of Fame coach*

---

Set a good example by showing respect for yourself, for them, and for others—opponents, parents, officials. You cannot demand respect. True respect must be earned.

## SUMMARY OF COACHING GUIDELINES

### Reacting to Athlete Behaviors and Competition Situations

*Good Plays and Effort*

*Do*: Provide *reinforcement!* Do so immediately. Let the athletes know that you appreciate and value their efforts, and reinforce effort as much as you do results. Look for positive things, reinforce them, and you will see them increase. Remember, whether athletes show it or not, the positive things you say and do remain with them.

*Don't*: Take their efforts for granted.

### Mistakes

*Do*: Give *encouragement* immediately after mistakes. That's when the youngster needs your support the most. If you are sure the athlete knows how to correct the mistake, then encouragement alone is sufficient. When appropriate, give *corrective instruction*, but always do so in an encouraging manner. Do this by emphasizing not the bad things that just happened, but the good things that will happen if the athlete follows your instruction (the *why* of it). This will make the athlete positively self-motivated to correct the mistakes rather than negatively motivated to avoid failure and your disapproval.

*Don't*: *Punish* when things are going wrong! Punishment isn't just yelling. It can be tone of voice, action, any indication of disapproval. Athletes respond much better to a Mastery Approach. Fear of failure is reduced if you work to reduce fear of punishment. Indications of displeasure should be limited to clear cases of lack of effort; but even here, criticize the lack of effort rather than the athlete as a person.

*Don't*: Give corrective instruction in a hostile, demeaning, or harsh manner. That is, avoid *punitive instruction*. This is more likely to increase frustration and create resentment than to improve performance. Don't let your good intentions in giving instruction be self-defeating.

### Misbehaviors, Lack of Attention

*Do*: Maintain order by establishing clear expectations. Emphasize that during competition, all members of the team are part of the activity, even those on the bench. Use reinforcement to strengthen team participation. In other words, try to prevent misbehaviors by using the Mastery Approach to strengthen their opposites.

*Don't*: Get into the position of having to constantly nag or threaten the athletes in order to prevent chaos. Don't be a drill sergeant. If an athlete refuses to cooperate, deprive him or her of something valued. Don't use physical measures, such as running laps. The idea here is that if you establish clear behavioral guidelines early and work to build team spirit in achieving them, you can avoid having to repeatedly *keep control*. Remember, youngsters want clear guidelines and expectations, but they don't want to be regimented. Try to achieve a healthy balance.

> The behavioral guidelines contained in the *Mastery Approach to Coaching* are easy to learn and to use.

### Getting Positive Things to Happen and Creating a Good Learning Atmosphere

*Do*: Give *technical instruction*. Establish your role as a caring and competent teacher. Try to structure participation as a learning experience in which you are going to help the athletes become the best they can be. Always give instruction in a positive way. Satisfy your athletes' desire to improve their skills. Give instruction in a clear, concise manner and, if possible, demonstrate how to do skills correctly.

*Do*: Give encouragement. Encourage effort, don't demand results. Use encouragement selectively so that it is meaningful. Be supportive without acting like a cheerleader.

*Do*: Concentrate on the activity. Be "in the competition" with the athletes. Set a good example for team unity.

*Don't*: Give either instruction or encouragement in a sarcastic or degrading manner. Make a point, then leave it. Don't let "encouragement" become irritating to the athletes.

## 5

# Communication and Self-Awareness

## *Skills for Improving Coaching Effectiveness*

As a coach, you are giving a great deal of time and energy to provide a worthwhile life experience for children. By putting to use the basic principles described in chapter 4, you can increase the positive impact you have on young people's lives.

A complete understanding of the Mastery Approach guidelines is essential for their effective use. In addition, communication skills and self-awareness are important for successful application of the guidelines.

### COMMUNICATING EFFECTIVELY

Everything we do communicates something to others. Because of this, develop the habit of asking yourself (and at times, your athletes) how your actions are being interpreted. You can then evaluate whether you are communicating what you intend to.

> Constantly ask yourself what has been communicated to athletes and whether the communication is effective.

Effective communication is a two-way street. By keeping the lines of interaction open, you can be more aware of opportunities to have a positive impact on athletes. Fostering two-way communication does not mean that athletes are free to be disrespectful toward you. Rather, it invites athletes to express their views (both positive and negative) with the assurance that they will be heard by you. Furthermore, by presenting a model of an attentive listener, you can hopefully improve the listening skills of your athletes.

Effective communication also requires that you view a team as a group of individuals and respond to these individuals accordingly. For example, a youngster who has low self-confidence may be crushed (or positively affected) by something that has no impact whatever on an athlete with high self-esteem. By improving your sensitivity to the individual needs of athletes, you can be more successful. The ability to "read" athletes and respond to their needs is characteristic of effective coaches at all levels.

## INCREASING SELF-AWARENESS

An important part of self-awareness is insight into how we behave and come across to others—knowing what we do and how others perceive what we do. One of the striking findings from our research—in which we observed and recorded actual coaching behaviors—was that coaches had very limited awareness of how frequently they behaved in various ways. Fortunately, awareness is something that can be increased. Two behavioral change techniques are recommended, namely, behavioral feedback and self-monitoring.

> As a coach, you occupy an important role, and increased awareness can help improve your effectiveness.

### Behavioral Feedback

Try to develop procedures that will allow you to obtain feedback from your assistants. In other words, work with assistant coaches as a team and share descriptions of each other's behaviors. You can then discuss alternate ways of dealing with problem situations and athletes and prepare yourself for handling similar situations in the future. Obviously, this requires an open relationship between coaches, a willingness to exchange feedback that may not always be positive, and a sincere desire to improve the ways in which you relate to athletes. Finally, at times, you may wish to discuss situations with your athletes to obtain feedback from them. This will show your athletes that you are interested in their reactions and are motivated to provide the best possible experience for them.

### Self-Monitoring

Self-monitoring (observing and recording one's own behavior) involves taking some time after practices and/or competitions to evaluate your behaviors and actions. When going through this self-analysis, ask yourself what you did relative to the suggested behaviors in the Mastery Approach guidelines. To assist you in this procedure, the box below presents a brief form for self-monitoring of desirable Mastery Approach coaching behaviors.

# COACH SELF-REPORT FORM

Complete this form as soon as possible after a practice or competition. Think about what you did, but also think about the kinds of situations in which the actions occurred and the kinds of athletes who were involved.

1. When athletes made good plays, approximately what percentage of the time they occurred did you respond with *reinforcement*? _____ %

2. When athletes gave good effort (regardless of the outcome), what percentage of the time did you respond with *reinforcement*? _____ %

3. About how many times did you reinforce athletes for displaying good sportsmanship, supporting teammates, and complying with team rules? _____

4. When athletes made mistakes, approximately what percentage of the time did you respond with

   a. Encouragement only? _____ %

   b. Corrective instruction given in an encouraging manner? _____ %

   (Sum of a plus b should not exceed 100%)

5. When athletes made mistakes, did you stress the importance of learning from them? _____ Yes _____ No

6. Did you emphasize the importance of having fun while practicing or competing? _____ Yes _____ No

7. Did you tell your athletes that doing their best is all you expect of them? _____ Yes _____ No

8. Did you communicate that winning is important, but working to improve skills is even more important? _____ Yes _____ No

9. Did you do or say anything to help your athletes apply what they learned today to other parts of their life (for example, doing the right things in school, family, or social life)? _____ Yes _____ No

10. Something to think about: Is there anything you might do differently if you had a chance to coach this practice or competition again?

# III

# PERFORMANCE ENHANCEMENT SKILLS FOR YOUNG ATHLETES

# 6

# Goal Setting

## Charting the Road to Success

Coaches and athletes are well aware that achieving one's potential depends on both skill and motivation. Skill and motivation are, of course, related. Athletes who are not motivated to develop their skills will probably not achieve their potential.

Motivation involves striving for particular goals. Thus, success as an athlete, as a coach, and as a team depends in large part on goal setting. Coaches must have goals. Teams must have goals. Individual athletes must have real, vivid, living goals. Goals help keep everyone on target. Goals commit athletes and coaches to the work, time, pain, and whatever else is part of the price of achieving success.

---

Transforming potential into performance involves setting and attaining goals.

—*Hubert "Hubie" Brown, Basketball Hall of Fame coach*

---

Coaches at all competitive levels are finding that specific goal-setting programs can have dramatic positive effects on both motivation and skill development. Their experiences are mirrored in the results of more than 100 scientific studies of goal-setting programs in business and industry. In over 90 percent of these studies, measurable increases in performance resulted when goal-setting procedures were introduced. Psychologists have learned a great deal about how to design and carry out effective goal-setting programs. By making use of these principles, you can increase motivation, performance, and the amount of fun and enjoyment that your athletes experience.

## WHY GOAL SETTING WORKS

There are many reasons why goal setting improves performance:

- Goal setting focuses and directs one's activities. Goals direct the athlete's attention and action to important aspects of the task. For example, a basketball player who sets a goal of increasing her free throw shooting percentage to 80 percent will concentrate on shooting free throws during practice time rather than taking many different kinds of shots.
- Goals help athletes mobilize effort. Returning to our basketball player, by setting this specific goal, she will likely exhibit greater effort and commitment in attempting to achieve this objective.
- Goals not only increase immediate effort but also increase persistence. As a case in point, the boredom of a long season is offset and persistence is increased when a golfer sets a number of short-term goals throughout the year.
- Athletes often develop and use new strategies for improving performance. For example, a baseball batter may change the mechanics of his swing in order to achieve a goal of hitting a certain percentage of line drives. Thus, setting and trying to attain specific goals may help increase motivation, commitment, and performance.

## HOW TO USE GOAL-SETTING PROCEDURES

Not all goal-setting procedures are created equal. Some approaches to goal setting are more effective than others. Research on the effectiveness of various types of goal-setting strategies suggests several practical guidelines.

1. *Set specific goals in terms that can be measured.* Specific goals are more effective in improving performance than are general "do your best" goals or no goals at all. Telling an athlete to "do as well as you can" does not make clear exactly what the person is to do. Therefore, it is essential that, in the athletic environment, goals be expressed in terms of specific measurable behaviors. Thus, setting goals in terms of specific free throw shooting percentages or number of turnovers is far more effective than encouraging players to "improve your free throw shooting" or "handle the ball better."

> Specific goals allow athletes to see exactly
> where they stand in relation to the goal.

2. *Set difficult but realistic goals.* Difficult or challenging goals produce better performance than moderate or easy goals. The higher the goal, the higher the performance, as long as the goal does not exceed what the athlete is capable of doing. Goals should not be so difficult that the athlete will fail to take them seriously or will experience failure and frustration in meeting them. It is therefore important for you to set goals in relation to each athlete's ability. The goals should be set so that they are difficult enough to challenge athletes but realistic enough to achieve.

3. *Set short-range as well as long-range goals.* Breaking down any long-term goal into smaller, more attainable goals leads to achievement and success. Short-range goals are important because they allow athletes to see immediate improvements in performance and thereby enhance motivation. Without short-range goals, athletes can lose sight of their long-range goals and the subgoals needed to attain them.

> Yard by yard it is awfully hard,
> but inch by inch it becomes a cinch!

One way to understand the relationship between short- and long-range goals is in terms of a staircase. The top stair represents the athlete's long-range goal or objective, and the lowest stair is his or her present level of performance. The steps in between represent a progression of short-term goals of increasing difficulty that lead from the bottom to the top of the stairs. The short-term goals allow athletes to enjoy successes and accomplishments as they move toward the top of the stairs.

4. *Set performance goals as opposed to outcome goals.* As we noted in chapter 2, our society places tremendous emphasis on the outcome of athletic events, and it is not surprising that many athletes are accustomed to setting only outcome goals such as winning or beating a particular opponent. The problem with outcome goals, however, is that athletes have only partial control over them. An athlete may achieve the best performance of his or her life and yet fail to achieve the outcome goal of winning an event because someone else performed even better. It is far better to set goals in terms of personal performance standards, for then success is seen in terms of athletes exceeding their own goals rather than surpassing the performance of others. When winning (outcome) becomes secondary to achieving personal goals, athletes are much more motivated to practice. Practices give athletes the opportunity to work toward their personal goals with assistance from the coach. Athletes do not judge themselves as having succeeded or failed purely on the basis of whether they have won or lost, but in terms of their achievement of the specific performance and behavioral goals they have set. Thus, the amount of personal satisfaction that athletes achieve from sport does not need to be tied to winning. Athletes at all levels of ability can enjoy success through attainment of their personal goals. Stating goals in such terms also helps athletes learn the valuable lesson that winning has more to do with *doing their best* than *being the best.*

---

Our goal is not stated in terms of winning, since that is not something we control, but rather, to execute as best we can.

—*Tom Osborne, College Football Hall of Fame coach*

---

5. *Express goals in positive rather than negative terms.* In line with the *Mastery Approach to Coaching* discussed in chapter 4, it is best to set goals in positive terms (number or percentage of plays carried out correctly) rather than in negative terms (number or percentage of mistakes made). This positive goal-setting procedure helps athletes focus on success instead of failure.

6. *Set goals for both practices and competition.* It is just as important, if not more so, to set goals for practice sessions as it is for competitive events. Practices are the times when athletes develop and hone their skills. When practice becomes meaningful as a result of being tied in with specific goals, athletes become more involved in what is going on, and practice time can be used much more productively. Moreover, setting specific goals related to practice and tracking progress toward them help reduce the drudgery of practice and makes it more meaningful for the athlete. During practice, each athlete can work toward specific performance goals that are geared to his or her areas of strength and weakness. Thus, one football player's goals may be keyed to improving his blocking, while another's may relate to tackling.

---

The will to prepare is the key to winning. You've got to pay the price. You play like you practice.

—*Johnny Majors, College Football Hall of Fame coach*

---

Since the presumed goal of every competitor is to win, it might seem meaningless to set additional goals during competition itself. However, such goals can be very useful in that they provide one means by which winning will be achieved. For example, a basketball team can set a team goal for a game, such as holding the opponent's best player to 15 points, outrebounding the other team, or limiting turnovers to no more than 10. By focusing on the attainment of specific performance goals, coaches can create a "game within the game" in which athletes can be successful in some important respects, even if they are not victorious in terms of the final score. Many coaches have found that this technique helps prevent players from being discouraged if the team does not win and helps promote steady improvement in the team's play.

7. *Identify specific goal achievement strategies.* All too often, goals are not accomplished because athletes fail to identify and commit themselves to goal achievement strategies. Setting goals without identifying ways of achieving them is not very effective. Thus, a basketball player who wants to improve his free throw percentage by 5 percent may choose an achievement strategy of shooting 30 additional free throws after practice each day.

8. *Record goals, achievement strategies, and target dates for attaining goals.* Once (a) specific goals have been set, (b) achievement strategies have been decided upon by the athlete and coach, and (c) target dates for goal accomplishment have been established, these should be written down so that they can be referred to frequently. Some coaches actually establish a formal contract with players to keep them focused on the activity and committed to it.

9. *Set up a performance feedback or goal evaluation system.* Goal-setting research indicates that performance feedback is absolutely necessary if goals are to enhance performance. Therefore, athletes must receive feedback about how their present performance is related to both short- and long-range goals. Without such feedback, athletes cannot track their progress toward goals and may be unable to see improvement that is actually occurring.

---

The best way to build confidence in your players is to show improvement through statistics.

—*Don James, College Football Hall of Fame coach*

---

Feedback can also correct misconceptions. Athletes, like other people, often have distorted perceptions of their own behavior. Objective evidence in the form of statistics or numbers can help correct such misconceptions and may help motivate corrective action. For example, it can be a sobering experience for a basketball player who fancies herself a great ball handler to find out that she has more turnovers than assists.

Feedback also creates internal consequences by causing athletes to experience positive (or negative) feelings about their performance. An athlete who is dissatisfied with his or her level of performance will experience feelings of self-satisfaction that function as positive reinforcement when subsequent feedback indicates improvement. The feelings of pride and self-confidence that arise can be even more important than external reinforcement from the coach in bringing out improved performance. Promoting self-motivation in athletes also reduces the need for coaches to reinforce or punish. When feedback is public, as in the posting of statistics, the actual or anticipated reactions of others can serve as an additional motivator of increased effort and performance.

10. *Goal-setting programs are most effective when they are supported by those individuals who are important in the athlete's life.* This typically includes the coach, teammates, and the athlete's family. Therefore, it is important that you promote the recognition, encouragement, and support of individual and team movement toward goals. You yourself are a central figure in providing such support.

### COMMON PROBLEMS WITH GOAL SETTING

In addition to the goal-setting principles presented above, there are some things to avoid. It is not particularly difficult to set up a goal-setting program. However, the preceding guidelines suggest some ways in which problems can arise when goal-setting procedures are used. One such problem occurs when too many goals are set too soon. If too many goals are set, athletes cannot properly monitor performance, or they find it very difficult to do so. A much better procedure is to rank the goals and focus attention on the one or two goals that are most important.

A second problem arises in setting goals that are too general. We have emphasized the importance of setting specific, measurable goals. The general principle here is that if you can't measure the goal in terms of specific numbers, it is too vague and general to be used effectively. Also, it is important to remember that performance goals are preferable to outcome goals because the athlete has greater control over them.

> Problems with goal setting are not difficult to overcome.

Finally, you may encounter athletes who have very negative attitudes toward goal setting and do not want to participate in such a program. It is best not to force such athletes to participate. More often than not, they will observe the benefits and enjoyment that other athletes are experiencing as a result of goal setting and will come on board.

## SETTING UP YOUR PROGRAM

To be successful in carrying out a goal-setting program, coaches must employ some sort of goal-setting system or procedure. The simplest and most effective system has three main phases: (a) the planning phase, (b) the meeting phase, and (c) the follow-up or evaluation phase.

### The Planning Phase

Setting up a goal-setting program obviously requires a good deal of planning on your part. First of all, you must identify individual and team needs. These may be in a variety of areas including performance, conditioning, sportsmanship, care of equipment, relations among teammates, and so forth. Once the most important of these are decided upon, you must decide how you can help your athletes achieve these goals. In other words, you yourself must engage in a goal-setting program in terms of identifying goals and specifying how you are going to help athletes attain them.

> Goal setting requires commitment on the
> part of the coach as well as the athletes.

### Meeting with Athletes

After goals have been decided upon, it is important that the coach communicate these to the athletes and indicate why they are important. How detailed you get in this meeting will of course depend upon the level of maturity of your athletes. With older and more experienced athletes, you may choose to meet with each one individually after the general meeting in order to mutually decide upon goals and strategies. For younger athletes, team rather than individual goals may be more appropriate, but it is essential that these goals be very specific and measurable.

It may be necessary to involve athletes in the measurement of behaviors relating to specific goals. For example, an athlete who is not currently playing in a soccer match may keep track of the number of passes made before each shot, if one of the goals is to work the ball around the defense before shooting.

### Follow-Up/Evaluation

In order to ensure that movement toward goals and possible revision of goals can occur, it is a good idea to set up several evaluation meetings with individuals, subgroups of athletes, or the entire team. A critical part of the entire process is the feedback procedure that you choose to employ. The procedure should allow you and your athletes to clearly see where things stand in relation to the goals that have been set. If your athletes are mature enough, you might require that they monitor their own target behaviors to supplement whatever statistics you might use to chart progress toward goals.

When coaches help athletes set realistic goals and provide ways for them to attain those goals, youngsters inevitably experience more success and feel more competent. By becoming more competent, they gain in self-confidence and become less fearful of failure. Perhaps most importantly, they discover that commitment to goals helps lead to success. They also learn, with your help, that failure indicates that they should try harder, not that they are unworthy. Deemphasizing winning and emphasizing attainment of personal and team goals can greatly increase the positive impact that a coach can have on the athlete's performance and enjoyment of the sport.

# 7

# Athletic Stress

## *Teaching Coping Skills to Young Athletes*

Sports challenge us. They place demands on us. The athletic setting is one in which we can test the limits of our abilities in competition with both ourselves and others. Many times, we are required to put ourselves on the line and to test our mental as well as physical limits.

These features of the sport environment not only attract people to sports, but they also serve as potential sources of stress. The physical and mental tests that are opportunities and challenges to some can be psychological threats to others. As we noted earlier, some athletes have a positive drive to succeed, and they regard pressure situations as challenges and rise to the occasion. Others, unfortunately, are motivated primarily by a fear of failing. When faced with the pressures of athletic competition, they are likely to be paralyzed by their fear and to choke.

The differences that exist in the ability of people to cope successfully with stressful situations are learned primarily during the childhood and adolescent years. Athletics can be an important arena in which such skills are learned. In a sense, the athletic experience can be a sort of laboratory for trying out and mastering ways of dealing with stress.

**WHAT IS STRESS?**

We typically use the term *stress* in two different but related ways. First, we use the term to refer to *situations* in our lives that place physical or psychological demands on us. Secondly, we use the term to refer to our mental, emotional, and behavioral *responses* to these demanding situations. These responses include such emotions as tension, anxiety, anger, and depression.

In the diagram, we present an analysis of stress that takes both the situation and the athlete's reactions into account. As you can see, four major elements are involved.

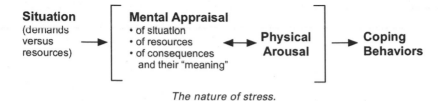

The nature of stress.

The first element is the external *situation* that is making some sort of physical or psychological demand on the person. Typically we view our emotions as being directly triggered by these pressure situations. This, however, is not the case. The true emotional triggers are not in the external situation, but in our minds, in what we have called *mental appraisal*. This evaluation process has several parts. First of all, we appraise the nature of the situation and the demands it is placing upon us. At the same time, we appraise the resources that we have to deal with it. We judge, in other words, how capable we are of coping with the situation. We also judge the probable consequences of coping or failing to cope with the situation and the meaning of those consequences for us.

The emotional responses that we call stress are likely to occur when we view ourselves as incapable of coping with a high-demand situation that has potentially harmful consequences for us. In response to such appraisals, our body becomes *physically aroused*, with pounding heart, rapid breathing, elevated blood pressure, tight and trembling muscles, and so on. This is part of the body's natural defense system, and it mobilizes us to respond to the emergency.

> The stress response includes negative thoughts, unpleasant
> feelings, and attempts to cope with the stressful situation.

The fourth element in our analysis of stress involves the *behaviors* that we use in order to try to cope with demands of the situation. Responses may be mental, as when a quarterback tries to figure out which play to call; they may be physical, such as shooting a free throw; or they may be social responses, such as dealing with an angry opponent.

### HOW STRESS AFFECTS YOUNG ATHLETES

Fear and anxiety are the emotions that are most frequently experienced as part of the athletic stress response. These are unpleasant states that most people try to avoid. There is evidence that this is precisely what many stress-ridden young athletes do. Avoiding or dropping out of sports is one of the ways some children escape from an activity they find threatening rather than pleasant.

In addition to influencing decisions about entering and/or continuing to participate in sports, competitive stress can detract from athletes' enjoyment of sports. Instead of a challenging, fulfilling activity, sports can become a threat to self-esteem and can rob children of the pleasures they should derive from participation. Eventually, this can take its toll on the athlete and produce burnout. Burnout is a legitimate concern, because burned-out athletes often show depression and a loss of drive and energy that carries over into other areas of their lives.

Stress affects not only how athletes feel, but also how they perform. All of us have seen athletes fall apart or choke under high levels of stress. When arousal is absent or extremely low, athletes frequently describe themselves as "flat" and do not perform as well as they are able. Some degree of arousal is usually needed for good performance. But at extremely high levels, arousal begins to interfere with performance. Research has shown that the more complicated or difficult the task, the less arousal it takes to interfere with performance. High-stress athletes who cannot control their emotions are likely to experience higher-than-optimal levels of arousal and perform poorly. The failure experiences that result only serve to reinforce these athletes' fears and undermine their confidence even more. Thus, a vicious circle involving anxiety, impaired performance, and increased anxiety can result. In pressure situations, high-stress athletes have difficulty concentrating and thinking clearly. This also serves to interfere with performance. Many young athletes never succeed in achieving their potential in sports because of their inability to control their anxiety.

> There is an optimal level of arousal beyond
> which performance begins to suffer.

Stress can affect physical well-being as well as performance. The physical nature of the stress response taxes the resources of the body and appears to increase susceptibility to illness and disease. Disruption of youngsters' eating and sleep patterns can occur. This is surely a high and unnecessary price to pay for the pursuit of athletic excellence!

Finally, research has shown that stress is related to an increased likelihood of athletic injury. Sports medicine specialists have also observed that athletes who find participation stressful and unpleasant often appear to take longer to recover from injuries. It may be that in some cases, an athlete finds in an injury a temporary and legitimate haven from the stress of competition.

We see, then, that stress can have many effects on athletes of all ages and that most of these effects are negative. Thus, athletes who develop coping skills that allow them to bear up under the pressure of competition, to be mentally tough in the face of athletic challenge and adversity, have a definite advantage.

## THE NATURE OF MENTAL TOUGHNESS

One of the highest compliments that can be paid to an athlete is to be labeled "mentally tough." Coaches speak of mental toughness as if it were a quality that a person either has or does not have. In reality, however, mental toughness is not something we are born with; rather, it is a set of specific, learned attitudes and skills.

The specific skills that constitute what we call mental toughness fall within the brackets of the stress model described above. Mentally tough athletes mentally appraise themselves and pressure situations in ways that arouse a positive desire to achieve rather than a fear of failure. Freedom from the disruptive effects of fear of failure allows them to concentrate on the task instead of worrying about the terrible things that will happen if they fail in the situation. Another specific skill that contributes to mental toughness is the ability to keep physical arousal within manageable limits. Somehow, these athletes are able to "psych up" with enough arousal to optimize their performance without being "psyched out" by excessive arousal. What mental toughness amounts to, therefore, is specific ways of viewing the competitive situation and skills relating to self-control of emotion and concentration.

> Mental toughness is a set of specific, learnable skills.

The core of mental toughness is the ability to control emotional responses and concentrate on what has to be done in pressure situations. The mentally tough athlete is in control of his or her emotions and is calm and relaxed under fire. Such athletes do not avoid pressure; they are challenged by it. They are at their best when the pressure is on and the odds are against them. Being put to the test is not a threat, but another opportunity to achieve. Mentally tough athletes are able to concentrate on the task at hand in situations where less capable athletes lose their focus of attention. They rarely fall victim to their own or others' self-defeating thoughts and ideas, and they are not easily intimidated. Finally, they are mentally resilient and have the ability to bounce back from adversity, their determination to succeed coming across as a quiet self-assurance.

It is no accident that mentally tough athletes tend to get the most out of their physical ability. Their level of performance seems to be more consistent, and they have a tendency to perform at their best when pressure is the greatest.

> Mental toughness can give a youngster the winning edge in sports, and in other life settings as well.

As a coach, you are in a position to help your young athletes develop the skills that comprise mental toughness. In doing so, you can help sports serve as a catalyst in their personal development.

## REDUCING STRESS AND BUILDING MENTAL TOUGHNESS

### Fear of Failure: The Athlete's Worst Enemy

Aside from fears of physical injury that produce stress for some athletes, most athletic stress arises from the fact that sport is an important social situation. The athlete's performance is visible to everyone present, and it is constantly being evaluated by the athlete and by significant people in his or her life. Many athletes dread the possibility of failure and fear the disapproval of others. Some feel that their athletic performance is a reflection of their basic self-worth, and they therefore have a great need to avoid failing. They are convinced that failure will diminish them in their own eyes and in the eyes of others.

We are convinced that fear of failure is the athlete's worst enemy. The thinking of high-stress athletes is dominated by negative thoughts and worries about failing. Unchecked, these concerns with failure undermine confidence, enthusiasm, the willingness to invest and persist, and, most importantly, the athlete's belief in himself or herself. It is these thoughts that transform the competitive athletic situation from what should be a welcome challenge to a threatening and unpleasant pressure cooker. It is these thoughts that not only cause concentration problems but also trigger the high physical arousal that interferes with performance.

> Fear of failure underlies most instances
> of choking under pressure.

The ideas that underlie fear of failure do not arise in a vacuum. They almost always have been communicated to youngsters by their parents or by other important adults, including coaches. This is not surprising, because the basic beliefs underlying such ideas are very widespread and accepted in our culture, which emphasizes achievement as a measure of personal worth. In our society, an untold number of children fall victim to their parents' demands that they perform exactly as expected, and to their parents' condemnations when they fail. Too often, the child's achievements are viewed as an indication of the worth of his or her parents, and failure brings reprisals based on the parents' feeling that they are to blame or that they themselves are inadequate. For many children, love becomes a premium handed out on the basis of *what a child can do* rather than simply *who he or she is.*

> Fear of failure is easy to create but hard to get rid of,
> because it is reinforced by widely accepted cultural beliefs.

The fastest and easiest way to create fear of failure in an athlete is to punish unsuccessful performance by criticizing it or by withholding love from the youngster. Under such circumstances, children learn to dread failure because it is associated with punishment or rejection. They also learn to fear and avoid situations in which they might fail. The unfortunate lesson they learn is that their worth and lovability depend on how well they perform. Instead of trying to achieve in order to reap the built-in rewards of achievement and mastery, children strive to perform well to avoid failure. They begin to measure themselves by their performance, and if their performance is inadequate, they usually consider their total being inadequate. A child can ultimately become so fearful of failing that all attempts to succeed are abandoned. This almost guarantees that the child cannot meet the standards he or she has set, and it serves only to reinforce feelings of inadequacy.

---

Because they fear failure, many people never try and thereby rob themselves of opportunities to be successful.

—*John Wooden, Basketball Hall of Fame player and coach*

---

Even though you enter into the life of a young athlete for a limited period of time, you can, as a coach, have a dramatic impact in helping the youngster develop a positive desire to achieve rather than a fear of failure. Earlier, we described four elements in the stress cycle: (a) the situation, (b) mental appraisal of the situation, (c) physical arousal, and (d) coping behaviors. Coaches can influence all four of these elements in ways that reduce stress and build mental toughness.

**Reducing Situational Stress**

The first way you can reduce stress is to change aspects of the situation that place unnecessary demands on young athletes. We are all well aware that coaches and parents can create stress by their actions. Many young athletes experience unnecessary stress because adults put undue pressure on them to perform well. Coaches who are punishing and abusive to children can create a very stressful and unpleasant environment. Similarly, parents who yell at their children during competitions or withdraw their love if the young athlete lets them down can create a situation in which the youngster runs scared much of the time. Eliminating such actions by coaches and parents can reduce unnecessary stress.

The behavioral guidelines presented in chapter 4 can help you reduce stress and create a more enjoyable atmosphere. The Mastery Approach emphasized in the guidelines is specifically designed to counteract the conditions that create fear of failure. The same is true of the philosophy of winning discussed in chapter 3. By promoting this philosophy of winning through use of the behavioral guidelines, you stand an excellent chance of creating a competitive sport environment in which athletes can enjoy themselves, develop their skills in an atmosphere of encouragement and reinforcement, and experience positive and supportive relationships with their coach and teammates.

> Coaches can be either a source of stress
> or a buffer against its harmful effects.

One of the most important differences between the *Mastery Approach to Coaching* and the negative approach is the kind of motivation that they produce. In the negative approach, punishment and criticism are used liberally in an attempt to stamp out mistakes. This approach operates by creating fear of failing. In contrast, the Mastery Approach makes use of encouragement and reinforcement in an attempt to strengthen desirable behaviors. The motivation that this kind of an approach develops is a positive desire to achieve and succeed rather than a negative fear of making mistakes. Thus, while both approaches may result in improvements in performance, they do so for different reasons and they create different types of motivation. Under the Mastery Approach, athletes come to see successful performance as an opportunity to experience a reward. On the other hand, the athlete who has been coached by the negative approach comes to view successful performance as a way of avoiding punishment. It is not surprising that athletes coached with a Mastery Approach come to see pressure situations as challenges and opportunities, whereas those subjected to a negative approach see the same kinds of situations as threats.

Parents can, at times, be a significant source of stress for young athletes. As a coach, you may be in a position to help parents correct stress-producing behavior patterns. Ideally, you would like your athletes' parents to be reinforcing the attitudes and outlooks about competition that you are communicating through your words and actions. In chapter 10, we discuss some ways in which you can accomplish this goal.

**Increasing the Athlete's Resources: Skills and Social Support**

Stress is experienced when we perceive an imbalance between the demands of the situation and the resources that we have to cope with the demands. It follows that another approach to reducing stress is to increase the young athlete's resources. Two types of resources are very important: (a) the skills the athlete possesses, and (b) the amount of support the athlete receives from important people, such as the coach, teammates, and parents. In your role as coach, you are in a position to influence both classes of resources.

It is quite natural to feel insecure when we don't have the skills needed to cope with a situation. Many young athletes experience this insecurity when they first begin to learn a sport. As their athletic skills increase, they become better able to deal with the demands of the athletic situation, and their stress decreases. Thus, being an effective teacher and working with young athletes to improve their skills is one way that you can help reduce athletic stress. Here again, we strongly recommend the positive approach, since we feel this is the most effective way to teach skills and create a positive learning environment. As athletes become more confident in their abilities, they see themselves as more prepared to cope with the demands of the athletic situation.

> Athletic stress can be combated by mastery
> of sport skills and by ample social support.

Earlier, we discussed how the Mastery Approach can create better relationships among coaches and athletes. Our research as well as studies of team building have shown that coaches who use this approach have more cohesive teams on which players like one another more. By using your own "reinforcement power" to encourage teammates to support one another, you help create a higher level of social support for all of your players. When a team can pull together and support one another in pressure situations, this kind of social support can help reduce the level of stress experienced by individual athletes.

### Developing Winning Attitudes toward Competition

Earlier, we noted that the term *stress* is used in two different ways. One use of the term relates to *situations* that place high demands on us. The other refers to our *response* to such situations. The importance of this distinction becomes particularly clear when we deal with the role of mental processes in stress. There is a big difference between *pressure situations* and *feeling pressure*. Mentally tough athletes perform well in pressure situations precisely because they have eliminated the pressure. They report that, although intellectually they are aware that they are in a very tough situation, they really don't feel the pressure on the inside. There is no way to eliminate pressure situations; they will always be there because they are a natural part of competition. This does not mean, however, that athletes have to respond to such situations by experiencing high levels of stress and getting psyched out.

Mentally tough competitors manage pressure well largely because they have become disciplined thinkers. Either consciously or unconsciously, they have made the connection in their own heads between what they think and how much pressure they feel during competition. They have learned (often the hard way) that thoughts like these produce pressure:

- "What if I don't do well?"
- "I can't blow it now."
- "I can't stand this pressure."
- "I'll never live it down if I lose."
- "If I miss these free throws, what will everyone say?"
- "If I don't sink this putt, I'll lose everything!"

On the other hand, mentally tough athletes think like this in pressure situations:

- "I'm going to do the best I can and let the cards fall where they may."
- "All I can do is give 100 percent. No one can do more."
- "This is supposed to be fun, and I'm going to make sure it is."

- "I don't have to put pressure on myself. All I have to do is focus on doing my job the best I know how."
- "I'm going to focus on the good things that will happen when I make the play."
- "I'm concentrating on performing, rather than winning or losing."

The first set of statements causes an athlete to react to adversity with bitterness, frustration, and anxiety. The second set of statements focuses attention where it should be—on giving maximum effort and concentrating totally on what has to be done. Pressure situations become welcome opportunities, rather than dire threats for mentally tough athletes. The bottom line is that the fundamental difference between mentally tough athletes and "chokers" is the way they choose to construct the situation in their heads. Situations are not nervous, tense, or anxious—people are! The sooner you can help athletes realize that pressure comes from within and not from outside, the sooner they can start shutting it down.

---

When an athlete can start loving adversity, I know I've got a competitor!

—Al McGuire, Basketball Hall of Fame coach

---

One of the great benefits of sports as a training ground for mental toughness is that the consequences of failure are temporary and unlikely to have a long-term impact on the future of a child (as failing in school might). This places you in an ideal position to help your young athletes develop a healthy philosophy about achievement and an ability to tolerate failure and setbacks when they occur. The starting point for such training is the philosophy of winning described in chapter 3. Great coaches develop mentally tough athletes and teams by realizing that an obsession with winning is self-defeating because it places the cart before the horse. They realize that effort should be directed not toward winning but toward performing to the very best of the athlete's ability at the time. Doing the very best one can at any moment should always be the focus and the goal. Winning will take care of itself; the only thing that can be directly controlled is *effort*. Mental toughness arises in the realization "I am competing against myself, not someone else. I will always be my own toughest opponent, and winning the battle with myself paves the way for winning the competition with my opponent."

Here are some specific attitudes that can be communicated to athletes by a coach.

1. *Sports should be fun.* Emphasize to your young athletes that sports and other activities in life are enjoyable for the playing, whether you win or lose. Athletes should be participating, first and foremost, to have fun.

2. *Anything worth achieving is rarely easy.* There is nothing disgraceful about its being a long and difficult process to master something. Becoming the best athlete one can be is not an achievement to be had merely for the asking. Practice, practice, and still more practice is needed to master any sport.

---

The dictionary is the only place that success comes before work. Hard work is the price we must pay for success.

—*Vince Lombardi, Pro Football Hall of Fame coach*

---

3. *Mistakes are a necessary part of learning anything well.* Very simply, if we don't make mistakes, we probably won't learn. Emphasize to your athletes that mistakes, rather than being things to avoid at all costs, are stepping stones to achievement. They give us the information we need to adjust and improve. The only true mistake is a failure to learn from our experiences.

4. *Effort is what counts.* Emphasize and praise effort as well as outcome. Communicate repeatedly to your athletes that all you ask of them is that they give total effort. Through your actions and your words, show your athletes that they are just as important to you when trying and losing as when winning. If maximum effort is acceptable to you, it can also

become acceptable to them. Above all, do not punish or withdraw love and approval when they don't perform up to expectations. It is such punishment that builds fear of failure.

5. *Do not confuse worth with performance.* Help your athletes distinguish what they *do* from what they *are.* A valuable lesson for children to learn is that they should never identify their worth as people with any particular part of themselves, such as their competence in sports, their school performance, or their physical appearance. You can further this process by demonstrating your own ability to accept your athletes unconditionally as people of value, even when you are communicating that you don't approve of some behavior. Also, show your athletes that you can gracefully accept your own mistakes and failures. Show and tell them that as a fallible human being, you can accept the fact that, despite your best efforts, you are going to occasionally bungle things. If your athletes can learn from you to accept and like themselves, they will not unduly require the approval of others in order to feel worthwhile.

6. *Pressure is something you put on yourself.* Help your athletes see competitive situations as exciting self-challenges rather than as threats. Emphasize that they can choose how they want to think about pressure situations. The above attitudes will help them develop an outlook on pressure that transforms it into a challenge and an opportunity to test themselves and to achieve something worthwhile.

---

The real competitor relishes the toughest situations. He doesn't have a choke level—he has an enjoyment level. He knows few athletes get to compete for the biggest rewards, and he loves it.

—*Johnny Majors, College Football Hall of Fame coach*

---

7. *Try to like and respect your opponents.* Some coaches and athletes think that proper motivation comes from anger or hatred for the opponent. We disagree. Sports should promote sportsmanship and an appreciation that opponents, far from being the "enemy," are fellow athletes

who make it possible to compete. Hatred can only breed stress and fear. In terms of emotional arousal, fear and anger are indistinguishable patterns of physiologic responses. Thus, the arousal of anger can become the arousal of fear if things begin to go badly during competition.

---

Athletes who play in a generally relaxed environment where there's good will toward their opponents are less fearful and play better.

—*Tom Osborne, College Football Hall of Fame coach*

---

When athletes learn to enjoy sports for their own sake, when their goal becomes to *do their best* rather than *be the best*, and when they avoid the trap of defining their self-worth in terms of their performance or the approval of others, then their way of viewing themselves and their world is one that helps prevent stress. Such youngsters are success-oriented rather than failure-avoidant. They strive to succeed rather than to try to avoid failure. Coaches who impart these lessons to their young athletes give them a priceless gift that will benefit them in many of their endeavors in life.

**Controlling Arousal: Teaching Your Athletes Relaxation Skills**

Coaches increasingly recognize the importance of psychological as well as physical skills. Despite this recognition, however, coaches have been given little information on how to teach psychological skills. It is no accident, therefore, that coaches spend almost all of their time teaching their players techniques and strategies, while pretty much leaving the learning of psychological skills to chance.

One very useful psychological skill that athletes can be taught by their coaches is relaxation. Most athletes perform better when they are in a moderately relaxed state. As noted earlier, a moderate level of emotional arousal can psych athletes up to perform more efficiently. On the other hand, high levels of arousal can interfere with thought and behavior patterns. Few athletes can perform well when they are all tensed up as a result of high arousal.

> Arousal can be controlled with relaxation training.

The ability to remain calm in a stressful situation, or at least to prevent arousal from climbing out of control, is a useful stress management skill. Many athletes have found that they can learn to prevent or control high levels of tension through training in muscle relaxation skills. Because one cannot be relaxed and tense at the same time, voluntary relaxation gives athletes the ability to turn off or tone down tension. Although it is clearly a skill and must be learned through work and practice, most people can be trained to relax.

Relaxation training actually has two benefits. The first is the ability to reduce or control the level of arousal, but the second is equally important. In the course of relaxation training, people become more sensitive to what is going on inside their bodies and are better able to detect arousal in its beginning stages. When they can detect the early warning signs of developing tension, they can plug in their coping responses at an early stage before the tension gets out of control.

We have been training athletes in relaxation skills for many years. We have found that children as young as 5 or 6 years of age can be trained in relaxation, and they can then use these skills to reduce tension and anxiety. Our experience has been that children who learn this and other stress-coping skills (such as the attitudes described earlier) show a marked increase in self-confidence and are less reluctant to tackle difficult situations. They apply these skills not only in athletics but also in other important life situations.

> Mastering coping skills at an early age
> can benefit a youngster throughout life.

We now describe a training program that you can use to train your athletes (and yourself, if you wish) in relaxation skills. The approach that we describe involves training through a process of voluntarily tensing and relaxing various muscle groups. The goal is to learn voluntary relaxation skills while gaining increased sensitivity to body tension. We find that within about a week of conscientious training, most people can increase their ability to relax themselves and reduce tension.

If you wish to help your athletes learn relaxation, we recommend that you go through the exercises on your own several times to become familiar with the procedure. Then you can easily guide your youngsters through the exercises until they become familiar enough with them to practice without your help. Many coaches to whom we have taught these procedures use them regularly as part of their practice sessions.

We recommend that the relaxation exercises be practiced at least once a day and preferably twice a day until they are mastered. They can be carried out in chairs or on a fairly soft floor (that is, on a carpeted floor or gym mats).

Explain to your athletes why they are learning this procedure, and point out to them that many champion athletes have learned this skill. As you guide the athletes through the exercises, use a slow, relaxed tone of voice. Give the athletes plenty of time to experience the sensations, and make sure that they are doing the breathing part of the exercises correctly. The goal of the training is to combine relaxation, exhalation, and the mental command to relax repeatedly so that the athlete will be able to induce relaxation by exhaling and mentally telling himself or herself to relax.

---

Mentally tough athletes have the ability to relax themselves quickly, even in the heat of competition.

---

In our training procedure, we start by concentrating on the hands and arms; move to the legs, stomach and chest, back muscles, and neck and jaw; and finish up with the facial and scalp muscles. Here are the steps.

1. While sitting comfortably, bend your arms at the elbow. Now make a hard fist with both hands, and bend your wrists downward

while simultaneously tensing the muscles of your upper arms. This will produce a state of tension in your hands, forearms, and upper arms. Hold this tension for 5 seconds and study it carefully, then slowly let the tension out halfway while concentrating on the sensations in your arms and fingers as tension decreases. Hold the tension at the halfway point for 5 seconds, and then slowly let the tension out the rest of the way and rest your arms comfortably in your lap. Concentrate carefully on the contrast between the tension that you have just experienced and the relaxation that deepens as you voluntarily relax the muscles for an additional 10 to 15 seconds. As you breathe normally, concentrate on those muscles and give yourself the mental command to relax each time you exhale. Do this for seven to ten breaths.

If you train your athletes, here is a sample of how you can phrase the instructions when presenting this exercise.

Do you know what uncooked spaghetti feels like? [They'll tell you hard, dry, and brittle. You can even have a piece with you to demonstrate.] That's almost what our muscles are like when we're all tensed up. You can't play sports when your muscles are like that. Now, what does cooked spaghetti feel like? Yes, it's soft and supple, like our muscles are when they're relaxed. What we're going to do is to learn to make our muscles like cooked spaghetti so we can quickly get rid of tension and play relaxed.

We're going to start out with the arms and hands. What I'd like you to do while keeping your eyes closed is to bend your arms and make a fist like this. [Demonstrate]

Now make a hard fist and tense those muscles in your arms hard. Notice the tension and the pulling throughout your arm as those muscles stretch and bunch up like rubber bands. Focus on those feelings of tension in your arms and hands. They're like uncooked spaghetti—hard and stiff.

[After 5 seconds] Now slowly begin to let that tension out halfway, and concentrate very carefully on the feeling in your arms and hands as you do that. Now hold the tension at the halfway point and notice how your arms and hands are less tense than before but that there is still tension present.

[*After 5 seconds*] Now slowly let the tension out all the way and let your arms and hands become completely relaxed, just letting go and becoming more and more relaxed, feeling all the tension draining away as the muscles let go and become completely relaxed. And now, each time you breathe out, let your mind tell your body to relax, and concentrate on relaxing the muscles even more. That's good . . . just let go. Let those muscles become soft and supple, like cooked spaghetti.

2. Tense the calf and thigh muscles in your legs. You can do this by straightening out your legs hard while pointing your toes downward. Hold the tension for 5 seconds, then slowly let it out halfway. Hold the halfway point for an additional 5 seconds, and then slowly let the tension out all the way and concentrate on relaxing the muscles as completely as possible. Again, pay careful attention to the feelings of tension and relaxation as they develop. Finish by giving the muscles the mental command "Relax" each time you exhale (seven to ten times), and concentrate on relaxing them as deeply as possible.

3. Press the palms of your hands together in front of your chest so as to tense the chest and shoulder muscles. At the same time, tense your stomach muscles hard. As before, hold the tension for 5 seconds, then slowly let the tension out halfway and focus on the decreasing levels of tension as you do so. Hold again for 5 seconds at the halfway point and then slowly let the tension out completely. Again, do the breathing procedure with the mental command to deepen the relaxation in your stomach, chest, and shoulder muscles.

4. Arch your back and push your shoulders back as far as possible to tense your upper and lower back muscles. (Be careful not to tense these muscles too hard.) Repeat the standard procedure of slowly releasing the tension halfway, then all the way. Finish by doing the breathing exercise and mental command as you relax your back muscles as deeply as possible.

5. Tense your neck and jaw muscles by thrusting your jaw outward and drawing the corners of your mouth back. Release the tension slowly

to the halfway point, hold for 5 seconds there, and then slowly release the tension in these muscles all the way. Let your head droop into a comfortable position and let your jaw slacken as you concentrate on totally relaxing these muscles with your breathing exercise and mental command. (You can also tense your neck muscles in other ways, such as bending your neck forward, backward, or to one side. Experiment to find out the way that's best for you. Tense your jaw at the same time.)

6. While sitting in a totally relaxed position, take a series of short inhalations, about one per second, until your chest is filled and tense. Hold each for about 5 seconds, then exhale slowly while thinking silently to yourself, "Relax." Most people can produce a deeply relaxed state by doing this. Repeat this exercise three times.

7. Finish off your relaxation practice by concentrating on breathing comfortably into your abdomen (rather than into your chest area). Simply let your stomach fill with air as you inhale, and deepen your relaxation as you exhale. Abdominal breathing is far more relaxing than breathing into the chest.

As you guide your athletes through the exercises, you can practice them yourself. You will find relaxation very useful in your own life. It not only serves as a weapon against tension and stress, but it produces an enjoyable state in its own right.

# 8

# Mental Rehearsal

## Using the Mind to Program the Body

---

The night before a game, I lie down, close my eyes, relax my body, and prepare myself for the game. I go through the entire lineup of the other team, one batter at a time. I visualize exactly how I am going to pitch to each hitter, and I see and feel myself throwing exactly the pitches that I want to throw. Before I ever begin to warm up at the ballpark, I've faced all of the opposition's hitters four times and I've gotten my body ready for exactly what it is I want to do.

---

The speaker was Nolan Ryan, one of the greatest baseball pitchers of all time. Ryan firmly believed that the mental skills he had developed over the years were every bit as important to his success as his physical talent. Among those skills were (a) the ability to relax and maintain his concentration under even the most adverse conditions, and (b) the ability to program himself through mental rehearsal.

Mental rehearsal goes by a variety of names, including *visualization* and *imagery*. We prefer the terms *mental rehearsal* or *imagery* rather than *visualization* because mental rehearsal involves far more than simply seeing with the mind's eye. Effective mental rehearsal involves all of the senses, including feeling the activity of one's muscles as they perform the skill. Whatever term you prefer, however, there is no question that mental rehearsal is one of the most powerful techniques for programming the body to perform as you want it to.

Sport science research has shown that a combination of physical and mental practice is often more effective than physical practice alone.

People in all walks of life, including many great athletes, have used imagery to enhance their performance. Moreover, research has supported the claims of many athletes that imagery improves their performance. Scientific studies have shown that although physical practice is still the most effective single method for learning and improving an athletic skill, a combination of physical *and* mental practice is often more effective than physical practice alone.

All of us have had firsthand experience in ways that our imagination can affect our thoughts, feelings, and behavior. Going back to your own childhood, can you recall instances in which you experienced excitement by thinking about the gift you might receive for your birthday or Christmas? Can you recall an instance in which you experienced the "dreads" by anticipating something very bad that might happen to you? Can you remember imitating the skills and style of your sport heroes? In all of these instances, imagery was involved. To imitate a baseball hero, for example, you had to be able to imagine his batting stance, how he swung the bat, how he wound up and threw the pitch, or how he fielded his position before you could copy it. Perhaps you even put yourself in his place, performing the same actions on a Major League field situated in your mind.

Imagery training involves the *systematic* use of mental rehearsal to program oneself for improved performance. It can be used as a means of learning or perfecting a skill, preparing oneself for competition, maintaining one's skill level while recovering from an injury, or developing a game plan. Before describing how you can use this powerful tool to enhance your coaching effectiveness, let us consider the nature of imagery and how it works.

## HOW IMAGERY IMPROVES PERFORMANCE

How does imagery work? How can simply imagining an action lead to an actual improvement in performance? The answer is that when we learn or perfect a skill, tiny electrical circuits are established in the nervous system and in the muscles that perform the act. Thus, when athletes engage in sport movements, the brain is constantly transmitting impulses to the muscles for the production of the movements. The reason imagery works is that similar impulses occur in the brain and muscles when athletes imagine the movements without actually performing them. Electrical recordings from the brain and muscles suggest that the low-level firing of nerve and muscle cells creates in the nervous system and muscles a kind of blueprint to help the individual execute the movement later on. This is sometimes called "muscle memory."

> Mentally rehearsing a skill strengthens the electrical circuits in the brain that control its performance, giving the brain a more vivid blueprint for the activity.

Whether athletes actually perform movements or simply imagine performing them, performance circuits in the brain and muscles are activated and strengthened with repetition. Imagery may have special benefits for strengthening the performance blueprint. Indeed, scientific research has shown that a mixture of mental rehearsal and physical practice actually results in a higher level of subsequent performance on athletic tasks than does 100 percent physical practice.

We know that imagery is effective for older athletes, but what about for children and adolescents? Actually, there is reason to expect that it might be even *more* effective for children. Children tend to be more image-oriented in their thinking than are adults, whose thinking tends to be more verbal in nature. In other words, youngsters tend to have more active and vivid imaginations. Studies of hypnotizability have shown that children tend to have greater ability than many adults to get into the suggestions (many of which involve imagery, such as imagining that one's hand is getting heavier and can't be moved).

> Research has shown that child athletes can profit
> significantly from mental rehearsal of sport skills.

Sport psychologists are now capitalizing on the imagery abilities of children, and studies of imagery training with young athletes are appearing in the scientific literature. In one such study, carried out by Dr. Li-Wie Zhang and his coworkers, 7- to 10-year-old elite Chinese table tennis players watched videotapes of the world's best players and imagined themselves performing the same techniques for 6 minutes a day 3 times a week for 16 weeks. These children showed much larger performance gains than did equally skilled children who only watched the videotapes but did not practice imagery.

You do not have to be a sport psychologist to use imagery techniques with your young athletes. By introducing them to the powers of their mind's eye, you can teach them a performance enhancement approach that they can apply in virtually any area of their life.

## INTRODUCING THE POWER OF IMAGERY TO ATHLETES

Youngsters want to be physically active when they come to practice, so you have to demonstrate the importance of imagery and justify your use of it early on. Here's a fun demonstration that shows how imagining a movement can actually cause it to occur involuntarily.

Seat the athletes in a circle facing a bench. Seat several youngsters (chosen because they will take their task seriously) on the bench and hand each subject a 6-inch piece of string with a large paper clip attached to the end. The string should be held with the thumb and forefinger, with the elbow resting on the athlete's thigh so that the paper clip hangs like a pendulum between the knees. Tell the other youngsters to watch but to keep silent during the demonstration.

Tell the subjects that you would like them to keep their eyes closed and to imagine the string and paper clip as vividly as they can. Ask them to nod when they form a good image of the string. Then tell them to imagine that the paper clip is beginning to move slowly back and forth, from right to left. Tell them to continue to imagine that it swings back and forth, more and more. After awhile, you will observe that the paper clips actually begin to move, at least for some of the children. (When that happens, motion to the other children to remain silent.) Then suggest a new image: that the paper clip is now moving toward and away from the subject. You will find that this typically occurs as well. You can also suggest clockwise or counterclockwise circular movements. (When the other athletes observe what happens, they will want to try the demonstration too. You might want to arrange some time after practice for this so as to conserve time and maintain control over the proceedings.)

After the demonstration (which almost always works for the majority of the youngsters), you can introduce the idea that imagining and feeling a skill helps one perform it better. Tell them that many champion athletes use imagery regularly, and that they can use it too.

## INCORPORATING IMAGERY TRAINING INTO YOUR PRACTICES

Many coaches of high school, college, and professional athletes schedule a 10- to 15-minute imagery period into their practice sessions, during which athletes form vivid images of performing sport skills flawlessly or mentally prepare themselves for the situations they expect to encounter. With younger athletes, imagery sessions exceeding 5 minutes can tax the athletes' attention span. Thus, you need to have your imagery session well planned. A good time to do imagery is immediately after stretching or warm-ups.

> In order to profit from imagery training, the athlete must have the coach's guidance on exactly what to imagine and feel.

In developing and refining skills through imagery, the athlete must know precisely what to imagine or rehearse, and then must form images that involve not only visual images but also images of what the movements *feel like* in the muscles. In order to form the correct image, the athlete must have a model for what to do. This can be based on watching someone else perform the activity or on the athlete's memory of a correct performance in the past.

When athletes are learning a new skill, most coaches show them how to do the particular skill. For example, baseball coaches show and tell the athletes how the bat should be swung, how the glove should be positioned to catch the ball, or which base the ball should be thrown to. Sometimes they have athletes who have already mastered the skill demonstrate it, or they show pictures or videotapes depicting the skill. Any of these demonstrations can be the basis for imagery. After the skill is demonstrated, tell the athletes to close their eyes and to see and feel themselves performing the skill, emphasizing the specific elements they should focus on. At first, you can have them view themselves "from the outside," as if they were watching a videotape of themselves. Then, they should imagine it "from the inside," as they would actually experience it. Emphasize the importance of trying to feel the action as well as seeing it in their imagination. Have them imagine performing the activity four or five times. You can use other embellishments, such as seeing the action in slow motion. The main thing is that they get engaged in the imagery.

For strategic instruction, such as playing a particular defense or reacting to a specific competition situation, discuss with the athletes exactly what should be done, making sure that each knows his or her assignment. Then, have the athletes imagine themselves reacting in the desired way.

After the athletes have done the imagery, have them perform the actual skill and notice any differences between what they imagined (presumably, the correct way to perform the act) and their actual behavior. This can provide valuable information on which specific elements of the skill or strategy need more work in both imagery and action. This approach also helps train your athletes to problem-solve and make adjustments, a valuable life skill.

Encourage your athletes to practice imagery on their own, both to refine skills and to prepare themselves for competition.

The beauty of mental rehearsal is that it can occur anywhere. Thus, a young athlete can shoot 20 free throws or block 20 shots on goal in the mental arena of the mind. Once a particular image has been established, encourage your athletes to spend a few minutes doing the imagery on their own. You (and they) will be surprised at the extent to which this process can speed up skill development. You can work with each individual athlete within the goal-setting concepts described in chapter 6 and decide which skills should be the focus of imagery training.

The *Mastery Approach to Coaching* emphasized throughout this book applies to imagery as well as to coaching behaviors and goal setting. Images should always focus on the desired response, never on the undesired one. The reason is obvious: Imagining what one does *not* want to do actually programs the body to do just that. Thus, caution your athletes to always form positive images, and make sure your instructions during imagery do not contain "don't" elements. To experience why, see what happens when we tell you *not* to imagine a pink elephant right now. What image did you form?

## MENTAL PREPARATION FOR COMPETITION

As Nolan Ryan did, many elite athletes use mental imagery to prepare for competition. Encourage your young athletes to do the same. A few minutes before each competition, meet with your athletes and give them any last-minute instructions or reminders. Then have them close their eyes and relax by focusing on their breathing and mentally saying "Relax" to themselves as they exhale. After perhaps 30 seconds of relaxation, ask them to vividly imagine and feel what it will be like to perform the specific skills or strategies you have just discussed. This can help relax and focus your athletes on what you want them to do.

Encourage your young athletes to use imagery to prepare themselves for competition even before they come to the competitive site. These few minutes of imagery can pay dividends in terms of mental preparation for competition.

Finally, encourage your athletes to use imagery in other areas of their life as well. Imagery, used correctly, is a life skill that can enhance performance in school, in social and family situations, and in peer relationships. Skills can be refined and valuable planning can occur in the mind's eye.

# COACHING CHALLENGES AND HOW TO DEAL WITH THEM

# Working Effectively with "Problem Athletes"

## Turning Problems into Opportunities

The most effective coaches are those who recognize that, no matter how much they think in terms of the team, the team is made up of unique individuals. Many outstanding coaches have emphasized the importance of being able to relate to athletes as individuals, of gaining insight into what makes each athlete tick, and of using that knowledge to help the athlete get the most out of himself or herself.

The name of this game is flexibility. Being flexible does not mean having different rules for different athletes, any more than fairness means treating everyone exactly alike. Team rules must hold for everyone, or discipline and respect break down quickly. On the other hand, knowledge of and respect for the makeup of each individual can be a key to successful coaching.

Athletes come in all shapes, sizes, and personality types. Some are a joy to coach, while others create problems for themselves and other people. Most coaches have had one or more athletes they have found difficult to handle. Others have known athletes whose psychological makeup limited their capacity to enjoy their sport experience or to perform up to their potential.

Left unattended, conduct problems or emotional difficulties can affect the success and enjoyment of coach and athletes alike. This in itself would be sufficient justification for trying to do something constructive about them. But another, and equally important, reason for discussing these problems is that the experiences a young athlete has in sports can help undo previous life experiences that have led to the problems. A sensitive and informed coach can promote a sport experience that helps the athlete learn new attitudes and problem-solving skills that improve personal adjustment. We believe firmly that the demands of the sport environment, together with the efforts of a sensitive and caring coach, can help build character in a manner that few other settings can.

> Sports can be a growth experience for problem athletes, but dealing with these athletes requires additional knowledge, understanding, and patience on the part of coaches.

Although the job description of youth coach does not include the term *amateur psychologist*, most coaches come to realize sooner or later that they are, in part, exactly that. And the most effective coaches are darn good amateur psychologists in the sense that they know how to influence athletes in ways that help them grow as people, not just as skilled performers.

---

The most important part of Little League has nothing to do with baseball.

—*H. E. Pohlman, former Washington Little League District 8 administrator*

---

"Problem athletes" fall into a number of different groups. We will describe some of the more common types, together with the kinds of life experiences that are likely to have produced the problems. Then we will describe methods that have proven successful in dealing with and, hopefully, helping such athletes.

## THE UNCOACHABLE ATHLETE
One of the most frustrating problems to deal with is the athlete who resists coaching. Such athletes often will not listen to instructions or

follow them, or they insist on doing things *their* way. Sometimes their resistance is expressed as open defiance and insistence that they know better than you how things should be done. In other cases, their resistance is never openly expressed but comes out indirectly. They may nod as if they're listening to you, then go and do as they please. This kind of indirect resistance can be even harder to deal with than the direct kind.

> Resistance may be expressed as open defiance
> or as a more subtle doing as one pleases.

Uncoachable or resistant athletes are frequently acting out unresolved problems in dealing with earlier authority figures. They usually have had negative experiences with adults in power positions, such as parents or teachers, who have forced them to do things against their will. Or, especially in cases involving divorce, they may view themselves as having been deserted or betrayed by the authority figure. They now carry their scars and residue of anger into other relationships with authority figures and resist them. In other cases, resistance is a part of the normal adolescent pattern of testing limits and challenging authority as a part of establishing independence. This normal resistance can usually be overcome by setting clear and reasonable guidelines and showing that you are going to insist upon compliance.

The natural tendency is simply to confront resistant athletes and tell them to "shape up, or else." Sometimes this solves the problem, but it is best to do this only as a last resort, especially if you want to help the athlete resolve the underlying problem. When you react in this manner, you may be doing exactly what past authority figures did to create the problem. Moreover, the athlete may agree to shape up, only to begin resisting you in new, indirect ways.

In the long run, what will help the resistant athlete most is a relationship with an authority figure who is firm, yet caring and trustworthy. This may take some time if the underlying problem is a severe one. In the beginning, you may find it helpful to say something like, "I have a hunch you've had some problems with people in authority in the past, and that these problems are coming out in this situation. I hope you'll find me to be a different person than past ones, but that will take time. In the meantime, I expect you to do what you're supposed to just like everyone else, and the amount of playing time you get will depend on that. If you have a question about why we're doing something my way, feel free to ask me about it, but do so at a time and place that doesn't interfere with what we're about."

> The resistant athlete may need exposure
> to a firm but caring authority figure.

Like any other set of behaviors, "coachability" can be strengthened through reinforcement. Rather than taking the chance of increasing resistance by using punishment to try to force compliance, try using the Mastery Approach to get the desired behaviors. Set clear expectations and, rather than taking compliance for granted, recognize and reinforce it when it occurs: "Way to go. You did exactly what we're trying to get across. That's the way to listen and execute!" This kind of an approach makes you a different kind of authority figure than the ones the athlete may still be struggling against, and it helps build a positive rather than an adversarial relationship.

## THE SELF-CENTERED SPOILED BRAT

Another "coach's delight," these athletes are selfish and wrapped up in themselves. They care little about anything except what *they* can get from participating. They usually come across as very sincere and nice, but this is a phony front that they use to con other people into giving them what they want. They will also pit people against one another to achieve their selfish goals. Such athletes believe that team rules and expectations are for others, not for "special" people like themselves. Before long, they are violating rules, but they have a million excuses for doing so. Over time, it becomes clear that they are unwilling to put the team ahead of themselves and do not want to cooperate unless they get some personal glory out of it.

> Dealing with "problem athletes" requires additional knowledge, understanding, and patience on the part of coaches.

These athletes typically have one of two different life history patterns. Some of them have been babied and pampered all their lives. They have never had limits placed on their behavior—they could do no wrong. As a result, they've grown up in an unrealistic world in which they were the centerpiece. They have no reason to believe that their athletic experience should be any different.

Other egocentric athletes have had quite the opposite life experiences. They have grown up in families where no one cared about them. They have had to learn to get what they want for themselves. The name of the game is "looking out for Number One," and they have become quite adept at manipulating others in order to achieve their ends.

Regardless of which pattern of life experiences is responsible, these athletes have to be told in no uncertain terms that there are definable limits and punishments for breaking the rules. The spoiled brat needs to learn that no individual is more important than the team, and that team goals take priority over individual goals. There are no special favors. Those who fit the first pattern described above can be told in a straightforward manner that the sport situation may be different than others they've been in. Those of the second pattern, who tend to see life as "dog eat dog," may need to be dealt with more sternly. The message must be that the only way they are going to get what they want out of the sport experience is to take others' needs into account as well as their own.

No special deals. There's no way you can have a team concept if one player knows that another player is getting a little bit more.

—*Don James, College Football Hall of Fame coach*

The sport experience can be one in which self-centered athletes learn that life involves give as well as take, and that considerable satisfaction can come from being a part of something larger than themselves. For the formerly deprived athlete, it can be a situation where mutual concern and caring are experienced for the first time.

## THE LOW-SELF-ESTEEM ATHLETE

These athletes have an inferiority complex. Their poor self-image may be limited to one or a few areas of their lives, or they may feel generally inferior to others. In sports, this comes across as a lack of confidence in their abilities, a reluctance to try to get better, or a lack of assertiveness. When they experience setbacks, they tend to see them as more evidence that they are inadequate. When they do well, on the other hand, they do not take credit for it. They attribute success to outside factors, such as luck or poor performance by their opponent. This pattern of taking personal credit for failures but not for successes helps perpetuate their low opinion of themselves.

Such athletes have usually not enjoyed much success in the past, and often they have been made fun of or had their inadequacies pointed out to them. They compare themselves unfavorably with others who are more successful, and they often set standards that are unrealistic or impossible to meet. They get into a way of thinking that "If I'm not the best, I'm the worst." Because they feel inferior, they act inferior, or they try to get attention in ways that get them into more problems.

> Feelings of inferiority help breed inferior performance as a self-fulfilling prophecy.

This is one type of problem that can really be helped by the kind of philosophy of success that we have discussed throughout the book. Low-self-esteem people get that way partly because they focus almost entirely on external outcomes over which they may have little control. They need to learn that success comes from *doing your best* rather than *being the best.* The focus with such athletes needs to be on individual goal setting and improvement that they can take personal pride in, and on the communication of caring and the conviction that they are worthwhile people. The goal-setting and performance feedback approaches described in chapter 6 can be very helpful for such athletes, for they can clearly see the results of their efforts and can't write them off as being due to chance or luck. If you can help them learn to take pride in their efforts and their willingness to put themselves on the line, the sport experience can be a turning point for them. With time, their efforts will result in successes that increase their self-confidence.

The kind of team climate that you help create can be very important for low-self-concept athletes. Using the Mastery Approach yourself, and emphasizing to your athletes that you expect them to support and encourage their teammates, can promote a positive interpersonal environment that gives plenty of social support to everyone, from star to bench warmer. In such an environment, the athlete who lacks confidence can get the support needed to begin to revise an inferior self-concept. Remember to use your "reinforcement power" to strengthen the desired support behaviors when they occur initially. After awhile, they tend to occur on their own because they create positive outcomes for everyone involved.

## THE HYPERANXIOUS ATHLETE

These athletes become tense and psyched out in competition. They tend to be very inconsistent in their performance level and have a tendency to perform poorly in pressure situations. Many of them display great talent in practice situations, but they choke and fall apart in competition. They are also prone to use injuries as a way of avoiding the challenges of competition.

You will recognize this pattern as indicative of the high-fear-of-failure athlete discussed in chapter 7. As we indicated there, the most common cause of high anxiety is a previous history of punishment or criticism for failure outcomes and a failure to reinforce effort. As a result, they feel threatened by achievement situations.

At the core of this problem are feelings of lack of control over outcomes and emotional responses. Hyperanxious athletes feel that they cannot control their anxiety, nor can they control the possibility of failing. The key is to give them feelings of greater control over both. The first step is to get them to focus on effort, over which they have complete control, rather than outcome, over which they have limited control. This relates to the philosophy of winning that we discussed in chapter 3. These athletes need to know that they will be supported whether they win or lose, if they give all they have. Getting this idea across to athletes helps reduce anxiety about failure. They need to learn to separate self-worth from performance so they can enjoy the demands of competition.

---

I've never been afraid to fail. . . . If you run into a wall, don't turn around and give up. Figure out how to climb it, go through it, or work around it.

—*Michael Jordan, Basketball Hall of Fame player*

---

Another approach to helping overanxious athletes gain control is to teach the emotional control skills described in chapter 7. Athletes who feel a lack of control over their anxiety can gain a massive dose of self-confidence when they learn relaxation skills. Knowing that one can control nervousness and tension gives hyperanxious athletes new feelings of control and a better chance of performing up to their capabilities. Ability to control body and mind is the stuff of which mental toughness is made.

## THE WITHDRAWN-SUSPICIOUS ATHLETE

These athletes seem to avoid getting close to others, and it is hard to involve them in the team. They may actively avoid being involved in activities with the rest of the team. More than simple shyness seems to be involved; there is a sense that they are afraid of close relationships with others. Others sometimes react to them with hostility because they misinterpret their standoffishness as resulting from feelings of superiority and feel rejected.

This pattern of avoidance of closeness often results from having been deeply hurt in close relationships with people who were important to them. They may have been let down, rejected, or painfully exploited in the past. This resulted in a fear of getting close to others and risking the vulnerability that closeness creates. As much as they may wish they could get close, they find it safer to maintain a barrier against being hurt again.

This is not the kind of problem that goes away immediately. Simply saying "You can trust me" is not going to be enough. You will need to prove yourself again and again by passing "trust tests." Be very straightforward and completely honest. Don't try to say things to build up the athlete unless you can document them. Be supportive and encourage the athlete to interact with others, but do not force him or her to do so. The sport environment can be one in which this athlete can gradually test the waters of relationships and experience the camaraderie that is such an important part of athletics.

---

The successful person is one who finds an opportunity in every problem. Unsuccessful people find a problem in every opportunity.

—*Lou Holtz, College Football Hall of Fame coach*

---

Problems with athletes can take many forms, and we have touched upon only a few of the more common varieties. Dealing with such athletes can be a demanding task that tries the patience of a saint. There may be problems that are so disruptive that you have no choice but to exclude the athlete for the good of the program, or instances in which severe personality problems indicate the need for professional attention. You are certainly not expected to function as a professional psychotherapist, nor should you try to in the case of severe personal problems. But you may be able to create an athletic experience that can have a significant positive impact on athletes who come to you with a previous life history that has resulted in personal problems. What more could any youngster hope to derive from athletics?

# 10

# Coach-Parent Relationships

## *A Vital Link in Successful Youth Sport Experiences*

Two important sets of adults combine to have a tremendous impact on youth sports. They are, of course, coaches and parents. The relationships that exist between coaches and parents go a long way toward determining the quality of the experience that young athletes have. Therefore, your role in dealing with parents can be very important to the success of your program.

Through their cooperative efforts, many parents productively contribute to youth sports. Unfortunately, the negative impact that some parents have is all too obvious. Out of ignorance, they can undermine the basic goals of youth sports and rob youngsters of benefits they could derive from participation. We hope that as a coach, you will be able to channel parents' genuine concerns and good intentions in a way that supports what you are trying to accomplish. This chapter provides information to assist you in working effectively with parents, thereby increasing the chances of a desirable sport outcome for all concerned.

### PARENT OBLIGATIONS AND COMMITMENTS

When a child enters a sport program, the mother and father automatically take on some obligations. Some parents do not realize this at first and are surprised to find out what is expected of them. Others never realize their responsibilities and therefore miss opportunities to help their child grow through sports, or actually do things that interfere with their child's development.

> Parents often lack knowledge about their obligations to their child's sport program.

To begin with, parents must realize that children have a right to participate in sports. This includes the right to choose *not* to participate. Although parents might choose to encourage participation, children should not be pressured, intimidated, or bribed into playing. In one study, athletes who felt "entrapped" reported less enjoyment and lower intrinsic motivation and benefits from being involved in sports, and they were more likely to drop out of sports. Even more profound and long lasting are the effects that feeling forced can have on parent-child relationships. Just how profound is shown in this statement made by a 40-year-old man: "If it hadn't been for sports, I wouldn't have grown up hating my father."

In fulfilling their responsibility, parents should counsel their child, giving consideration to the sport selected and the level of competition at which the child wants to play. And, of course, parents should respect their child's decisions.

Sometimes the best decision is not to participate. Participation in sports, although desirable, is not necessarily for everyone. For children who wish to direct their energies in other ways, the best program may be no program. Many parents become unnecessarily alarmed if their child does not show an interest in sports—particularly if the parents themselves had positive sport experiences. They think that a child who would rather do other things must somehow be abnormal. But forcing a child into sports against his or her will can be a big mistake. Sometimes the wisest decision is to encourage the child to move into other activities that may be more suited to his or her interests and abilities, at least until an interest in sports develops.

Parents should be observers and supporters of their athletically inclined children, but never pushers.

—*Wayne Gretzky, Hockey Hall of Fame player*

Parents can enjoy their child's participation more if they acquire an understanding and appreciation of the sport. This includes knowledge of basic rules, skills, and strategies. As a coach, you can serve as a valuable resource by answering parents' questions and by referring parents to a community or school library or a bookstore for educational materials (books and videos). For example, a 45-minute self-instructional DVD titled the *Mastery Approach to Parenting in Sports* is designed to help parents create a mastery climate and thereby get coaches and parents on the same page. (Visit http://www.y-e-sports.com for a 12-minute video preview.) In addition, you might devote part of an early season practice to a lecture/demonstration of the fundamentals of the sport. Parents having little background in the sport should be encouraged to attend this session.

Some parents unknowingly become a source of stress to young athletes. All parents identify with their children to some extent and thus want them to do well. Unfortunately, in some cases, the degree of identification becomes excessive. The child becomes an extension of the parents. When this happens, parents begin to define their own self-worth in terms of their son's or daughter's successes or failures. The father who is a "frustrated jock" may seek to experience through his child the success he never knew as an athlete. The parent who was a star may be resentful and rejecting if the child does not attain a similar level of achievement. Some parents thus become "winners" or "losers" through their child, and the pressure placed on the child to excel can be extreme. The child *must* succeed or the parent's self-image is threatened. Much more is at stake than a mere competition, and the child of such a parent carries a heavy burden. When parental love and approval depend on how well the child performs, sports are bound to be stressful.

| Parents can be a potent source of athletic stress. |
| --- |

As a coach, you might be able to counteract this tendency by explaining the identification process to parents. Tell them that if they place too much pressure on a child, they can decrease the potential that sports can have for enjoyment and personal growth. A key to reducing parent-produced stress is to impress on them that youth sports are for young athletes, and that children are not miniature adults. Parents must acknowledge the right of each child to develop athletic potential in an atmosphere that emphasizes participation, personal growth, and fun.

To contribute to the success of your program, parents must be willing and able to commit themselves in many different ways. Seven key questions serve as thought-provoking reminders of the scope of parents' responsibilities. Parents should be able to honestly answer yes to each one.

### 1. Can the Parents Share Their Son or Daughter?

This requires putting the child in your charge and trusting you to guide his or her sport experience. Part of this requirement involves accepting your authority and the fact that you may gain some of the child's admiration and affection that the child once directed solely at his or her parents. This responsibility does not mean that parents cannot have input. But as the coach, you are the boss! If parents are going to undermine your leadership, everyone concerned is going to have problems.

### 2. Can the Parents Admit Their Shortcomings?

Parents must be convinced that the proper response to a mistake or not knowing something is an honest disclosure. For example, if their child asks a question about sports, and they do not know the answer, they should not be afraid to admit it. An honest response is better than a wrong answer. Coaches and parents alike should show children that they realistically accept whatever limitations they have. Surely nobody is perfect, but sometimes children do not learn this because adults fail to teach them.

**"Perfect" people simply do not exist.**

### 3. Can the Parents Accept Their Child's Triumphs?

Every child athlete experiences "the thrill of victory and the agony of defeat" as part of the competition process. Accepting a child's triumphs sounds easy, but it is not always so. Fathers, in particular, may be competitive with their sons. For example, if a boy does well in a competition, his father may point out minor mistakes, describe how others did even better, or remind his son of even more impressive sport achievements of his own.

### 4. Can the Parents Accept Their Child's Disappointments?

In addition to accepting athletic accomplishments ("the thrill of victory"), parents are called upon to support their child when he or she is disappointed and hurt ("the agony of defeat"). This may mean not being embarrassed, ashamed, or angry when their son or daughter cries after losing a competition. When an apparent disappointment occurs, parents should be able to help their child learn from the experience. By doing this without denying the validity of their feelings, parents can help their child see the positive side of the situation and thus change their child's disappointment into self-acceptance.

### 5. Can the Parents Give Their Child Some Time?

Parents need to decide how much time they can devote to their child's sport activities. Conflicts arise when they are very busy yet are also interested and want to encourage their child. To avoid this, the best advice you can give parents is to deal honestly with the time-commitment issue and not promise more time than they can actually deliver. Recommend that they ask their child about their sport experiences and make every effort to watch some of their competitions.

> Fulfilling parent obligations requires
> them to invest time in their children.

### 6. Can the Parents Let Their Child Make His or Her Own Decisions?

Accepting responsibility for one's own behavior and decisions is an important part of growing up. You should encourage parents to offer suggestions and guidance about sports, but ultimately, within reasonable limits, they should let the child go his or her own way. All parents have ambitions for their child, but they must accept the fact that they cannot dominate the child's life. Sports can offer an introduction to the major parental challenge of letting go.

### 7. Can the Parents Show Their Child Self-Control?

Parents should be reminded that they are important role models for their child's behavior. It is not surprising to find that parents who lose control themselves often have children who are prone to emotional outbursts and poor self-discipline. Coaches can hardly be expected to teach sportsmanship and self-control to youngsters whose parents obviously lack these qualities.

> Youngsters learn from what they see.

## PARENT BEHAVIOR AT SPORT EVENTS

As part of their responsibilities, parents should watch their child compete in sports. Fortunately, the majority of parents behave appropriately at youth sport events. But the minority who misbehave can spoil it for all the rest. It takes only a few inconsiderate parents to turn what should be a pleasant atmosphere into one that is stressful for all concerned.

Coaches, program directors, sport officials, and the athletes themselves have a right to demand that spectators conform to acceptable standards of behavior. Youth sport authorities recommend six rules for parental behavior:

1. *Do* remain seated in the spectator area during the event.
2. *Don't* interfere with the coach. Parents must be willing to relinquish the responsibility for their child to the coach for the duration of the practice or competition.
3. *Do* express interest, encouragement, and support.
4. *Don't* shout instructions or criticisms to the child.
5. *Do* lend a hand when a coach or official asks for help.
6. *Don't* make abusive comments to athletes, parents, officials, or coaches of either team.

These rules make good sense. There is also a video rule that is easy to remember. When parents attend practices and competitions, they should imagine they are being videotaped. The two-part rule is simple:

- *Don't* do anything that would embarrass yourself or your child.
- *Do* things that would make your son or daughter proud.

What about parents who violate the rules of conduct? When parents misbehave, it is the duty of program administrators, sport officials, and other parents to intervene. It is not your *primary* job! You have a huge responsibility in taking care of the team and cannot be expected to police the spectators as well. This perspective must be qualified for the sport of soccer. The rules of youth soccer specify that coaches are responsible for the behavior of parents. Because of this, the most effective approach is for coaches to enlist the assistance of parents. In other words, coaches should delegate authority to parents. They should be asked to step in and correct inappropriate behavior when they see or hear it.

## PROMOTING TWO-WAY COMMUNICATION
There is a difference between genuine concern for one's child and disruptive meddling or interference. Parents have both the right and the responsibility to inquire about *all* activities that their child is involved in, including sports. They should take this responsibility seriously,

probing into the nature and the quality of specific sport programs. By so doing, they are not being overly protective or showing a lack of confidence in you or your program. Rather, they are fulfilling a child-rearing obligation to oversee the welfare of their loved one.

Tell parents of your willingness to discuss any problems that might arise. Let them know that you are open to receiving their input. Also, remember that productive exchange cannot occur unless there is an atmosphere of mutual respect and courtesy.

If you keep the lines of communication open, you will be more likely to have constructive relations with parents. There is, however, a proper time and place for interaction with you. That time is not during practice or competition, and it is never in the presence of the youngsters. Tell parents what times and places are best suited for discussions with you.

---

**Communication is the key to friendly, productive relations with parents.**

---

Certain children may have specific characteristics that you should know about. For example, they may have medical or psychological problems that could affect their participation. Encourage parents to share this type of information with you on a confidential basis. This will help prepare you to deal more effectively with the young athlete, and perhaps with the parents as well.

Perhaps the most common cause of coach-parent conflicts is a difference of opinion about the young athlete's abilities. In this regard, the use of a performance measurement system (described in chapter 6) not only provides valuable feedback to athletes but can be an objective source of performance evaluation for parents. Nevertheless, sometimes parents will disagree with what you are doing as a coach. The main thing is not to get defensive. Even if you do not agree, you can at least *listen* and evaluate the message. You might find some of their suggestions helpful. In the end, however, *you* are the coach and have the final say. Remember that no coach can please everyone. No one can ask any more than what you ask of your athletes—doing the very best job you can and always looking for ways to improve.

## DEALING WITH "PROBLEM PARENTS"

Most parents are enthusiastic and have a true concern for their child. Sometimes, however, parents simply do not realize the trouble they are causing. Instead of being angry with them, recognize that they have a problem—one that you can help solve. Your task is to point out to these people, tactfully and diplomatically, the negative influences of their actions and encourage them to become more constructive and helpful. Some common types of "problem parents" are described below, together with recommendations for dealing with them.

### Disinterested Parents

*Distinguishing Characteristics*

The most noticeable characteristic of disinterested parents is their absence from team activities to a degree that is upsetting to their child.

*What You Should Do*

Try to find out why the parents do not participate and contribute, and let them know that their involvement is welcome. Make sure you avoid the mistake of misjudging parents who are actually interested but have good reasons (work, sickness, etc.) for missing activities. Explaining the value of sports and how they can draw children and parents closer together may provide parents with a new interest in the activities of their child. In this situation, the athletes need help too. You should encourage them and show that you are really interested in them as people.

*What You Can Say*

"Ms. O'Rourke, Danny is showing tremendous improvement, and he really enjoys playing soccer. If you attended a few practices or games, you could make it an even better experience for him. Is there anything you can do to make this happen?" *Or* "Ms. O'Rourke, I know parents are very busy, but it would be fantastic if you could attend some of our practices or games. That would really make Danny feel great! Do you think you can free up some time for this?"

## Overcritical Parents

### Distinguishing Characteristics

Overcritical parents often scold and berate their child. Such parents are never quite satisfied with their child's performance. They give the impression that it is more their experience than it is the athlete's.

### What You Should Do

As discussed earlier, some parents unconsciously equate the success or failure of their child with their own success or failure. As a result, they are often hard on their child. You should attempt to make overcritical parents aware of this problem as tactfully as possible. Explain how constant criticism can cause stress and emotional turmoil for their youngster—irritation that actually hinders performance. Tell them why you prefer to use praise and encouragement to motivate and instruct young people, and how parents can do the same.

### What You Can Say

"Mr. Jones, I know you're only trying to help Nathan, but when you criticize him, he gets so nervous that he plays worse, and that certainly takes any fun out of it for him." Or "Mr. Jones, I've found that Nathan responds much better to encouragement and praise than he does to criticism. If you were to encourage your son instead of criticizing him so much, sports would be a lot more enjoyable for both of you. After all, it's the kids' game. They play for fun, and too much criticism spoils it for them."

## Parents Who Scream from behind the Bench

### Distinguishing Characteristics

Some parents seem to have "leather lungs" and large vocal cords. They often sit directly behind the bench, which makes them a distinct danger to the well-being of your eardrums. They frequently rant and rave and virtually drown out everyone else speaking in the area, including you. Everyone is the target for their verbal abuse—team members, opponents, coaches, sport officials.

*What You Should Do*

Do not get into an argument with a screaming parent. It will not do any good and will probably make things worse. During a break in the competition (half time, between periods), calmly, tactfully, and privately point out to the person that such yelling is a poor example for the young athletes. You can ask other people to help out by working with this person during competitions. Also, you can give the disruptive parent a job that will help the team (scouting opponents, keeping stats, looking after equipment, etc.). This may provide a greater sense of responsibility and help the screamer keep quiet. If the screaming persists, seek assistance from administrators.

*What You Can Say*

"I know it's easy to get excited, but these kids are out here to have a good time. Try not to take the game so seriously, okay?" *Or* "Listen, why don't we get together after the game and you can give me some of your ideas on coaching? I'd rather have them afterward because during the game, they're very confusing."

**Sideline Coaches**

*Distinguishing Characteristics*

Parents who assume the role of sideline coaches are often found leaning over the bench making suggestions to athletes. They may contradict your instructions and disrupt the team.

*What You Should Do*

Again, do not confront such a parent right away. Advise your athletes that during practices and competition, you are the coach and that you want their full attention. Listening to instructions from others may become confusing. Tell the parent privately how confusing it is for the athletes when two or more people are telling them what to do. You might ask the parent to be either a full-time assistant coach or a full-time spectator.

### What You Can Say

"Ms. Meadows, I appreciate your concern and enthusiasm for the team. But when you coach Nancy from the sidelines, it becomes confusing and distracting to her and the other kids. I know you've got some good ideas, and I want to hear them. But please, after the game."

### Overprotective Parents

#### Distinguishing Characteristics

Most often, the overprotective parents are the mothers of the athletes. Such parents are characterized by their worried looks and comments whenever their son or daughter is playing. Overprotective parents frequently threaten to remove their child because of the dangers involved in the sport.

#### What You Should Do

You must try to eliminate the fear of injury by reassuring the parent that the event is fairly safe. Explain the rules and equipment that protect the athlete. Point out how good coaching, program administration, and officiating add to the safety of the sport.

#### What You Can Say

"Ms. Taylor, we try to make the game as safe as possible for the athletes. You've got to remember that I wouldn't be coaching kids if I didn't care about them or if I thought the sport was dangerous for them." *Or* "Ms. Taylor, I care about each one of these kids, and I would never let any of them do anything that I thought would endanger them."

## CONDUCTING A COACH-PARENT MEETING

As a coach, you unselfishly devote a tremendous amount of time and effort to providing a worthwhile life experience for youngsters. All too often, you are asked to do "just one more thing." However, successful coaches are aware of the importance of securing the aid and support of well-informed parents. Rather than facing the task of dealing with individual "problem parents" later, a preseason meeting can be the key to reducing the chance of unpleasant experiences. In other words, having a coach-parent meeting is well worth the additional time and effort!

> Having a preseason sport orientation meeting
> is a good investment for everyone.

This part of the chapter is a guide for planning and conducting effective coach-parent meetings. Because each coach is unique, it is recommended that you evaluate these suggestions and information and make modifications to suit your personal situation.

### Purposes of the Meeting

The overall objective of a coach-parent meeting is to improve parents' understanding of youth sports and what you are trying to accomplish. The following are some more specific purposes:

- To enable parents to become acquainted with you.
- To educate parents about the objectives of youth sports and clarify the goals of your program.
- To inform parents about the specifics of the program and what is expected of the children and parents relative to these details. This includes obtaining parental assistance for accomplishing various tasks and conducting the season's activities.
- To get parents to understand and reinforce the *Mastery Approach to Coaching* that you will be using.
- To inform parents about their youth sport obligations and commitments.
- To establish clear lines of communication between you and parents.
- To help you understand the concerns of parents.

A coach-parent meeting might also be used to increase parents' knowledge of the sport. Information about basic rules, skills, and strategies is probably not necessary for the more popular sports but could be beneficial for the lesser-known sports. However, time limitations usually prevent their coverage at a coach-parent meeting. As suggested earlier, part of an early season practice could be devoted to a lecture-demonstration of sport fundamentals. Parents having little background in the sport should be encouraged to attend this session.

## Planning and Preparation

One reason for being hesitant about conducting a coach-parent meeting is that you might feel insecure about leading a group of adults. This is not unusual. People are often reluctant to do things for which they have had little training or previous experience. Coaches who have held meetings with parents indicate that it is not an overtaxing experience, and the benefits make the meeting a good investment. The meeting does not have to be elaborate to be successful. However, the importance of being well prepared and organized cannot be overemphasized!

> Leading a coach-parent meeting can be enjoyable.

### When Should the Meeting Be Held?

Schedule the meeting early in the season, preferably a week to 10 days before the first practice. A weeknight or Saturday morning is probably most convenient. This can be determined by talking with several parents to learn of their preference for the day, time, and place of a meeting.

### Where Should the Meeting Be Held?

Ideally, your league or club will have a central facility that could be used. If not, the location you select should be easily accessible and should have a meeting room of adequate size, with appropriate features (seating, lighting, etc.). If necessary, solicit the assistance of parents. For example, a businessperson might have access to a company conference room; a teacher might be able to secure the use of a schoolroom; or a service club member might have use of the club facility.

### How Long Should the Meeting Be?

It will take approximately 75 minutes to cover the necessary topics. It is your responsibility to start the meeting on time, keep it moving along, and finish reasonably close to the specified time.

### Should Athletes Attend the Meeting?

Some coaches have no objection to having athletes attend the meeting with their parents. They believe it helps improve communication among all those involved. Other coaches find it more productive to conduct the meeting without the athletes present. Your personal preference will determine the policy adopted. However, if you elect to exclude the athletes, make special arrangements for parents who might not be able to attend without their children. For example, an additional room might be sought in which the children could be shown an educational sport video under the supervision of an assistant coach.

### How Should Parents Be Informed about the Meeting?

Use a personal e-mail to notify parents. (Such information is typically provided as part of the registration process and appears on the team rosters that are made available to coaches.) This should be sent at least a week before the meeting date. Include brief statements about the objectives of the meeting, its importance, and the parents' responsibility for attending. Also include information about the date, time, location and directions, attendance by youngsters, and other specifics that you feel are necessary. Send a team roster, including e-mail addresses and telephone numbers, with the correspondence. As an additional way of promoting attendance, follow-up e-mails before the meeting are recommended.

*How Can the Content Be Organized?*

Provide parents with a written program outline. A carefully prepared outline improves the organizational quality of the meeting, and it helps parents understand the content. Following an outline makes it easier for you to keep the meeting moving in a crisp, systematic way. This serves to avoid wasteful time lags.

> You should develop your reputation as a well-organized leader.

*What Other Preparation Is Necessary?*

You might want to provide name tags. Name tags are a good way to learn identities, and they promote the friendly environment that is necessary for a successful meeting. Finally, having refreshments before and after the meeting (coffee and doughnuts, juice, etc.) is an effective way to promote interaction among the parents.

### Content and Conduct of the Meeting

For any educational program, even the best content is of doubtful value if the program leader does not establish a cooperative learning environment, or if the leader creates hostility and resistance. If you conduct your meeting as a two-way sharing of information, defensiveness and ill will can be minimized. Some of the parents in attendance will have a considerable amount of knowledge about sports. Therefore, it is best to take advantage of their expertise by encouraging them to share it with the group.

> Effective communication is a two-way street,
> requiring both speaking and listening skills.

As the leader of the session, you will do most of the talking. However, the meeting will be more effective if you involve the parents in a discussion, instead of lecturing them. You can do this by (a) encouraging parents to ask questions, and (b) directing questions to them from time to time and relating their answers to the main points you want to make. Also, in creating an open atmosphere for exchange, it is very important to show respect for the parents. Make them feel that they are a contributing part of the meeting, rather than a mere audience.

The coach-parent meeting described below contains seven separate components. The following program elements are included: (a) opening, (b) objectives of youth sports, (c) details of your sport program, (d) coaching roles and relationships, (e) parent obligations and commitments, (f) coach-parent relations, and (g) closing.

### Opening (5 minutes)

Begin the meeting by introducing yourself and your assistant coach(es). During the welcome, let the parents know that you appreciate their interest and concern. Some parents may not care enough to attend, but those who do attend deserve credit. In praising their dedication, point out that they are taking an important step toward assuring a quality sport experience for their child.

---

**Parents deserve praise for attending your meeting.**

---

In order to gain the parents' respect, your credibility must be established. You can do this by giving pertinent background information about your experience in the sport, your experience as a coach, and special training that you have had, such as attendance at coaching workshops and clinics. Let the parents know that you are a competent coach who will make every effort to provide a positive sport experience by doing the best job you can.

During this introductory period, identify the purposes of the meeting. In addition, you might want to invite parents to attend an early practice session. This will serve to provide them with information about fundamentals of the sport. It will also familiarize them with your coaching style.

A note of caution is in order. You might be conducting a coach-parent meeting for the first time or might have little experience in leading adults. Do not begin the meeting by announcing this as a personal shortcoming or by asking for the parents' tolerance. Such statements may reduce their trust in and support for you as their child's coach. Self-degrading remarks may also cause parents to question your ability to conduct the meeting. To gain respect, you must show confidence in leading the session.

### Objectives of Youth Sports (10 minutes)

After the opening remarks, there should be a discussion of the objectives of children's athletics, including a healthy philosophy of winning (see chapter 3). Focus on those goals that are a major part of your coaching. Also, find out which objectives the parents would like to have emphasized. As pointed out earlier, if coaches and parents work together to reduce misunderstandings, the objectives can be achieved.

> Youth sports provide a variety of educational
> opportunities for young athletes.

### Details of Your Sport Program (10 minutes)

During this part of the meeting, present details about the operation of your sport program. In addition to other items that you might think of, give consideration to the following:

- Equipment needed and where it can be purchased
- Sites and schedules for practices and competitions
- Length of practices and competitions
- Team travel plans
- Major team rules and guidelines
- Special rule modifications to be used at this level of competition
- Medical examinations
- Insurance
- Fund-raising projects

- Communication system for cancellations, etc.
- Midseason and postseason events

You should also provide information about what is expected of the athletes and parents relative to the program details. Some coaches find it useful to organize a parent committee, giving this committee the task of coordinating parent involvement in many activities of the season.

### Coaching Roles and Relationships (10 minutes)

Parents will benefit from knowing about your coaching style. In addition to describing the Mastery Approach that you will be using (see chapter 4), encourage parents to use this approach in interactions with their child.

> The *Mastery Approach to Coaching* emphasizes the use of reinforcement, encouragement, and sound technical instruction.

### Parent Obligations and Commitments (20 minutes)

Informing parents about their roles in youth sports and the responsibilities you expect them to fulfill is the most important part of the meeting. Discuss the following topics, which were covered earlier in this chapter:

- Counseling their child about sports selection and the level of competition at which they want to play—conferring with and listening to them
- Dangers of over-identification by parents with their child—the negative impact of this process
- Parent commitments—the seven important questions to which parents must be able to honestly answer yes
- Rules for parent behavior at competitions—as the coach, you are responsible for the team, and as parents, they are responsible for their own behavior

### Coach-Parent Relations (5 minutes)

Tell parents of your willingness to discuss any problems that might arise—remember, two-way communication! You should let them know what times and places are best suited for discussions with you.

### Closing (20–30 minutes)

We recommend concluding the meeting with a question-and-answer session. There is an effective technique for starting it. Specifically, you can take the lead in raising questions. Stimulate parent involvement by asking the first few questions, and then guide the discussion. If you do not know the answer to a question, do not be ashamed to admit it. The parents will appreciate your honesty. Rather than giving a weak or incorrect response, indicate that it is a question to which you can both seek an answer. Perhaps someone in the audience will be able to provide the answer. Do not give the impression that every question must be addressed and answered by you.

> You can serve as a valuable source
> of sport information for parents.

You might want to take some time to assess the format and content of the meeting and your style of presentation. Evaluative comments might be solicited from parents through informal discussion. Feedback can be valuable for making changes to improve the quality of future meetings. Finally, at the end of the meeting, do not forget to thank the parents again for attending.

The coach-parent meeting is a vitally important tool for developing parent involvement and support. A successful meeting will help solidify the athletic triangle (coach–athlete–parent) and lead to positive youth sport experiences.

# 11

# What to Do If . . .

During our *Mastery Approach to Coaching* workshops, we always allocate a period of time for discussion of challenging issues and situations that the coaches themselves have encountered. Over the years, certain critical issues have surfaced repeatedly, suggesting that there is a good chance that you, too, might have to deal with one or more of them. In this chapter, we present common problems and recommendations for solving them.

### SHOULD KIDS EVER BE CUT?

Heartbreak can be experienced when youngsters are eliminated from sports participation. Surely not all children can be on the team of their choosing, but we believe that every youngster should have a chance to play. Prior to the age of 14, the practice of cutting children from sport programs is indefensible. At the high school level it is appropriate to have select leagues to allow gifted athletes to develop their skills. But even at this age, alternative programs should be available for less talented youngsters who wish to play the sport.

The tragedy of cutting children from sport programs lies in the fact that those cut are almost always the least skilled or those who have discipline problems. It is precisely these children who are in need of an opportunity to grow through sport. Here again, we must choose between a professional model and one devoted to the development of children.

What should you do if you must cut a youngster? The first thing is to realize that whether or not the athlete shows it, he or she is likely to feel disappointed, rejected, and perhaps even humiliated. The youngster needs your support at this very difficult time. You can give support by acknowledging the disappointment felt by the child. Do not tell the child not to be disappointed or make unrealistic excuses for why it happened. All people must learn to face disappointments in life. You can make this easier if you show that your personal regard for the child has not diminished.

In addition to communicating your understanding, you may be able to suggest options in other programs in the same sport or in other sports. One child who was at first devastated by being cut from a peewee football team was helped by his coach to get involved in a soccer program and is now having a great time.

## WHAT IF AN ATHLETE WANTS TO QUIT?

At one time or another, and for a variety of reasons, most athletes think about quitting. Sometimes a decision to quit comes as a shock to the coach, but at other times the warning signs leading up to the decision are very clear.

What are the causes of dropping out of youth sports? In general, the reasons fall into two categories. The first category involves a shift in interests, especially in adolescents. Other involvements, such as a job, a boyfriend or girlfriend, or recreational pursuits may leave little time for sports involvement. In such cases a youngster may simply choose to set other priorities.

The second general set of reasons why youngsters drop out relates to negative sports experiences, such as the following:

- Not getting enough playing time
- Poor relationships with coaches or teammates

- An overemphasis on winning that creates stress and reduces fun
- Over-organization, excessive repetition, and regimentation, leading to boredom
- Excessive fear of failure, including frustration or failure to achieve personal or team goals

If the youngster has decided that other activities are more important, his or her priorities should be respected. However, it is wise to provide a reminder that a commitment has been made to the program and to teammates and that athletes owe it to themselves and to others to honor commitments and to finish out the season. This gives the youngster an opportunity to feel good about himself or herself by fulfilling the obligation through the rest of the season—even if the activity itself is no longer pleasurable.

If the decision to quit is based on one or more of the negative factors listed above, there is a legitimate problem that you as coach need to address. These problems are far less likely to occur when the *Mastery Approach to Coaching* principles have been applied. Indeed, as our research on the dropout issue has shown, the Mastery Approach is the best way to avoid such problems. If athletes begin dropping out, we recommend that you honestly examine your own coaching practices in light of the behavioral guidelines in chapter 4.

## UNUSUAL DISCIPLINARY PROBLEMS

In chapter 9, we discussed approaches to dealing with several classes of problem athletes. Although they may be a headache for the coach, most problem athletes can be successfully dealt with. Given our emphasis on the benefits of participation and our opposition to cutting athletes, are there ever instances in which an athlete should be expelled from a program?

Unfortunately, there are a few athletes whose behavior is so disruptive or even dangerous to others that the welfare of others must override the concern for the individual. For example, one coach discovered that a team member was offering drugs to other athletes. In another instance, a youngster was subject to uncontrollable violent outbursts against his teammates. Obviously, such behaviors cannot and should not be tolerated.

Elimination from a program is a last resort that should occur only after reasonable efforts have been made to correct the problem. The situation is complicated by the fact that sports may be the only medium for reaching the child, and your relationship with the youngster may turn out to be a curative one for a child from a bad home situation.

If you encounter an especially severe disciplinary problem, the first step may be a conference with the parent(s) to see if they can help. In some extreme cases, referral to a professional counselor may allow the child to remain in the program, and continued participation can be used to motivate change. In any event, it is not your responsibility as a coach to shoulder the burden alone, and it is not fair to subject your other athletes to intolerable situations. You have plenty to do as a coach; do not hesitate to seek outside assistance.

## WHEN INJURY PREVENTS PARTICIPATION

A young athlete may be temporarily eliminated from a sport program because of an injury. This may be less painful to the athlete's self-esteem than being cut, but it can in many ways be just as frustrating. One of the disappointments of being injured is that the youngster no longer feels a full part of the team.

You can counteract this by making sure that the athlete is included in team practices and competitions in some capacity. For example, an injured softball player can coach the bases and keep the scorebook.

Another constructive activity for the injured athlete is mental rehearsal. You can recommend that the athlete who cannot participate actively during practice do so by using imagery, and injured athletes should be encouraged to mentally practice their skills. Many injured athletes have reported that they maintained their skill level or even performed at a higher level when they returned because of the use of mental rehearsal.

## DEALING WITH A TOUGH LOSS OR LOSING STREAK

Children differ a great deal in their reactions to a loss. Some may be barely affected or may forget the loss almost immediately. Others will be virtually devastated by the loss and may be low-spirited for days. Avoid the temptation to deny or distort what the child is feeling. If one of your players has struck out three times and made an error that lost the game, she does not want to hear, "You did great." She knows she didn't, and your attempts to comfort her in this manner may well come through as a lack of understanding about how she feels. Likewise, it is not very helpful to tell a child, "It doesn't matter." The fact is that at that moment it does matter a great deal!

Is there anything you can do to make your athletes feel better without distorting reality? One thing you can do is to point out something positive that was achieved during the competition. A wrestling match may have been lost, but some good takedowns and escapes may have been executed. By emphasizing these accomplishments, you can help your athletes paint a more balanced picture.

Another thing you can do is to look to the future rather than dwell on the loss. Nothing can be done about the loss, so the most productive view is to focus on what has been learned and what can be used to improve future performance.

Above all, don't blame or get angry with the athletes if they have given maximum effort. They feel bad enough already. Support and understanding, sincerely given, will be very helpful at this time. If they haven't given maximum effort, communicate your unhappiness without disparaging them as people. They need to learn that effort is completely controllable and that they are accountable. Again, focus on the future and tell them that they owe it to themselves and their team to give maximum effort. Effort is a *decision*, not a trait.

Perhaps your team loses regularly. If winning is the only goal that is set, athletes will be constantly frustrated. If, on the other hand, goals focused on effort and improvement are emphasized, a sense of accomplishment can result as improvement occurs, and this can help blunt the disappointments of losing. Knowledgeable coaches often use individual and team goal setting to create a kind of "game within the game." For example, the team objective may be to reduce the number of errors, strikeouts, fumbles, or penalties in the next few games. Even if competitions are lost, children can experience a sense of accomplishment as they attain modified goals.

You can promote similar goal setting on an individual level with your athletes. In addition to performance goals, you can place emphasis on such important ingredients to success as effort and teamwork. Many a team and many an athlete has been helped to feel as if progress was made toward a larger objective when they succeeded at smaller subgoals.

## DEALING WITH A WINNING STREAK

Strangely enough, winning can create its own problems. One is overconfidence and the well-known swelled head. Unless carefully handled, winning teams can become arrogant and disrespectful to teams they defeat. And a long winning streak can provide pressures of its own when the emphasis becomes the outcome rather than the process of competition.

Youngsters should be allowed to feel good about winning—they've earned it. But they should also be reminded to show consideration for their opponents. Emphasize that it never feels good to lose and there is no justification for rubbing it in. Instead, tell youngsters to be gracious winners and to give their opponents a pat on the back or a handshake in a sincere manner. Remind them that their opponents make it possible for them to enjoy the process of competing.

During a winning streak, most athletes experience not only the pleasure of winning but also the increased pressure not to lose (especially when the parents jump on the bandwagon). An additional danger is that if a team wins too regularly and too easily, they may get bored and take their success for granted. A focus on effort and continued improvement can provide an additional and meaningful goal for youngsters. It is important to communicate that you expect continual striving for victory. Again, winning is to be sought, but it is not the only objective. Finally, don't allow your athletes to rest on past laurels. Point out that past success does not constitute a guarantee of no mistakes or losses in the future.

## TROPHIES AND OTHER AWARDS

Children usually participate in sports because of their intrinsic motivation to play for the fun of it. What happens when material or extrinsic awards, such as money and large trophies, are introduced as an additional reward for winning? Can children lose their intrinsic motivation? Sadly, the answer is yes.

If carried to an extreme, external rewards can replace intrinsic motivation as the reason for participating in sports. When young athletes begin to see these extrinsic rewards as the reason for their participation, the removal of these rewards may result in a loss of interest in participation.

An unhappy example of exactly this effect is the case of a teenage wrestler whose father called one of us. The father was very concerned because his young athlete refused to enter meets unless the winners' trophies were large enough to justify competing.

We are not suggesting that trophies and other extrinsic rewards be eliminated from sports. They certainly have their rightful place as a means of recognizing outstanding effort and achievement. It is important, however, that adults and children maintain a proper perspective so that trophies do not become the be-all and end-all of participation. It is sad indeed when children lose the capacity to enjoy athletic competition for its own sake. Make sure the awards are of modest proportion, and be sure to have awards for the most-improved and dedicated player, as well as the most skillful one.

## MISBEHAVIOR BY OTHER COACHES

Some of the knottiest problems that arise in youth sports involve relationships with other coaches. Sometimes coaches witness unacceptable behavior by other coaches that could have serious negative consequences for youngsters. The tricky part comes in deciding whether it is appropriate for you to be involved. When does appropriate concern become interfering and meddling? What should you do if issues like the following crop up?

- The coach is mistreating youngsters either verbally or physically.
- The coach is engaging in unacceptable behavior, such as bad language, inappropriate touching, or hazing of officials or opponents.
- The coach is using technically incorrect, questionable, or possibly dangerous coaching methods.
- The coach is losing perspective of the purpose of youth sports and seems preoccupied with winning, thus putting additional stress on athletes.

Because each situation is somewhat unique, there are no cut-and-dried answers that apply to every case. Nonetheless, there are some general principles that can be helpful in approaching and resolving such problems.

When incidents such as those listed above occur, it would be a mistake not to consider them problems. As uncomfortable as it may be to either confront or report another coach, we must never lose sight of the primary focus—the welfare of the children.

If you have a personal relationship with the coach that will permit you to approach him or her with your concerns, this can be a useful avenue to resolving the problem. On the other hand, it may be necessary to express your concerns to the program administrators, whose responsibility it is to take the appropriate remedial actions.

## CAN YOU BE SUED?

Part of our modern-day society includes an increased tendency for people to seek legal compensation for real or imagined wrongs. Anyone who occupies a position that can affect the welfare of children, including the youth coach, has a rightful (and legal) responsibility to provide a safe experience. A coach who fails to carry out this responsibility (either by acting irresponsibly or by failing to act responsibly) can be sued and found guilty of negligence.

Technically, a judgment of negligence requires that (a) you have a legal duty, (b) you failed to fulfill that legal duty, (c) someone to whom you owed the duty sustained an injury, and (d) your failure to fulfill the duty caused the injury. Under these conditions, you can be found guilty of negligence and be subject to substantial financial penalties.

During the past 30 years, an increasing number of lawsuits have been filed against youth sport coaches, and the court decisions in these cases have established nine legal duties of coaches. Awareness of these duties can help you carry out your responsibilities in a manner that enhances the welfare of young athletes as well as your ability to defend yourself against litigation.

### Duty 1. Plan the Activity Properly

Plan your practices and suit them to the current skill levels and physical conditioning of your athletes, allowing for individual differences. Do not practice advanced skills until your athletes are ready for them—they may be dangerous for unprepared youngsters. Likewise, adapt training regimens to the current conditioning level of your team.

In fulfilling your planning duty, you must:

- Develop a season-long plan that incorporates skill-appropriate teaching progressions
- Evaluate athletes to determine their skill levels and physical conditioning
- Write lesson plans for all practices
- Adjust your teaching progression to the individual characteristics of your athletes
- Closely follow your plans
- Keep records of your athlete evaluations and practice plans

## Duty 2. Provide Proper Instruction

Several sport techniques, such as spear tackling in football and head-first sliding in baseball, have been linked with a high risk of injury and deemed unsafe to use. Moreover, legal judgments against coaches have affirmed that such techniques should never be taught to young athletes or even permitted for them. You have a duty to teach technical and tactical skills correctly in accordance with accepted procedures of the sport, thereby reducing the likelihood of injury. This duty includes an obligation to learn safe teaching procedures via reading sport-safety literature, watching safety videos, and/or attending safety clinics.

In fulfilling your instructional duty, you must:

- Be knowledgeable about current instructional standards for your sport and apply them in your teaching
- Teach techniques, strategies, and rules according to accepted methods of your sport and the maturational level of your athletes
- Provide instructions in a clear, complete, and consistent manner, including adequate feedback on skill-learning progressions
- Closely supervise all instructional/practice and competition activities at all times, even when others are delegated a role of leadership

## Duty 3. Warn Athletes and Parents of Inherent Risks

Every sport has risks associated with it, and many legal suits have been based on the claim, "I was never warned that this could happen." Youth sport programs have tried to protect themselves by including discussions of foreseeable risks in parent orientation meetings and on parental consent forms. Likewise, athletes should be warned of foreseeable and potentially dangerous situations and taught what to do if they occur. The goal here is not to frighten parents and athletes unduly, but rather to give them a reasonable basis for decisions about assuming the risks inherent in the sport. To accomplish this, your warnings should be clear, thorough, and repeated.

In fulfilling your warning duty, you must:

- Warn athletes and parents of the inherent risks of the sport to enable them to know, understand, and appreciate the dangers of participation
- Use written notices, releases, videos, and repeated warnings to ensure the risks are fully comprehended

### Duty 4. Provide a Safe Sport Environment

As a coach, you are responsible for regularly and thoroughly inspecting the safety of the sport environment—the playing facility, plus warm-up, training, and dressing areas. This involves making sure there are no hazards, such as holes, broken glass, exposed sprinkler heads, or sharp corners. If there are hazards that you cannot remedy, you have a duty to (a) notify the facility manager that the environment is unsafe, and (b) warn your athletes about hazardous conditions and steer activity away from them as much as possible.

In fulfilling your environment-safety duty, you must:

- Regularly inspect the sport environment, noting and (whenever possible) remedying hazardous conditions
- Develop and regularly use a facilities-and-equipment inspection checklist, and keep completed checklists on file
- Correct dangerous conditions and/or reduce the hazards to the best of your ability; warn athletes of hazards; and notify the facility manager about them
- Give athletes safety rules; regularly remind them of the rules; and consistently enforce the rules
- Monitor the changing sport environment, and make prudent judgments about continued participation if conditions become hazardous

### Duty 5. Provide Adequate and Proper Equipment

Baseball bats with loose handgrips, hockey face masks incorrectly mounted in the helmets, or loose bolts in gymnastics equipment are examples of accidents waiting to happen. You are responsible for providing athletes with the best equipment in order to provide the greatest degree of safety. Courts have ruled that coaches must be diligent in the manner in which equipment is selected, distributed, used, and repaired. If equipment is used improperly, you can be held liable for any resulting injuries to athletes.

In fulfilling your equipment-safety duty, you must:

- Provide the best age/skill-appropriate equipment that reasonably can be afforded
- Teach your athletes how to properly fit, use, and inspect their equipment. Encourage them to return ill-fitting or defective equipment
- Inspect all equipment regularly for wear and tear, and ensure that it continues to comply with safety standards
- Allow only qualified people to install, fit, adjust, and repair equipment
- Warn athletes of potentially hazardous equipment, and give proper instructions on using it
- Keep up-to-date on accepted safety standards for equipment of your sport

### Duty 6. Match Your Athletes Appropriately

The responsibility here is to avoid placing youngsters at risk by matching them against others who are much larger, stronger, or physically skilled. This is particularly important in contact sports (e.g., football, soccer, wrestling), but it is also relevant in sports that involve throwing or striking balls. One-on-one contact drills between a 100-pound and a 200-pound football player reflects poor judgment on the coach's part and can be the basis for a judgment of negligence.

In fulfilling your matching duty, you must:

- Match athletes according to age, size, maturity, skill, and experience in order to avoid situations in which the risk of injury is increased
- Enforce rules designed to promote equitable and safe competition
- Avoid mismatches, but modify practices and drills to appropriately accommodate them when they do occur

- Make appropriate safety adjustments for mismatches associated with between-sex competition, athletes returning to participation after recovering from injury, and athletes with disabilities

### Duty 7. Evaluate Athletes for Injury or Incapacity

Another situation that can place an athlete at significant physical risk is health problems or a previous injury. Most programs require a pre-participation physical examination to ensure that athletes do not have a health problem or unhealed injury that could be dangerous. This responsibility also pertains to judgments of when an injured athlete can resume participation. One general guideline is that an athlete who has been knocked unconscious should not be allowed to return to action without receiving medical clearance. It should be noted that this duty is not yours solely. Rather, it is shared with parents, athletic trainers, and physicians who specialize in sports medicine.

In fulfilling your injury-evaluation duty, you must:

- Ensure that each athlete's health is satisfactory for participation at the beginning of the season
- Determine whether an illness or injury is sufficiently threatening to warrant discontinuation of participation in practice or competition
- Ensure that injured athletes are fully recovered before allowing them to return to play

### Duty 8. Supervise the Activity Closely

As a supervisor, you are in charge of your athletes and assistant coaches. Supervision has two separate but related levels. The basic requirement for *general supervision* is to maintain visual and auditory contact with the area and individuals under supervision, and to be able to respond quickly. In addition to the sport playing area, examples of areas in which general supervision is required include locker, shower, and equipment rooms; bleachers; hallways; and stages adjacent to a gymnasium.

*Specific supervision* is instructional in nature and directed toward the actual teaching or coaching of an activity. It occurs at the immediate location of an activity and is more action oriented than general supervision. In general, (a) the more dangerous the activity is, the more specific the supervision should be, and (b) more specific supervision is required with younger athletes and less experienced athletes. Supervision is a learned skill, and a qualified supervisor is a person who has adequate education and certification to appropriately perform instructional tasks.

In fulfilling your supervisory duty, you must:

- Provide general supervision for athletic facilities and playing areas your team uses
- Provide specific supervision when teaching new skills and when the risk of injury increases
- Know your sport well enough so you can anticipate potentially dangerous situations and be able to proactively remedy them
- Use informational posters, notices, and signs to supplement your supervision
- Prohibit reckless or overly assertive behavior that threatens the well-being and/or safety of any athlete

### Duty 9. Provide Appropriate Emergency Assistance

Coaches have a responsibility to provide or secure appropriate medical assistance for injured athletes. If appropriate medical assistance is not immediately available, coaches have the duty to provide immediate and temporary care. Therefore, training in first aid and CPR must be available to coaches on an annual basis. When an injury occurs, you should provide only the first aid you are qualified to perform, and transfer the risk associated with emergencies to more qualified people. After an injury, you should complete an injury-report form.

In fulfilling your emergency-assistance duty, you must:

- Obtain a consent form from each athlete at the beginning of the season
- Protect injured athletes from further harm

- Provide immediate and appropriate first aid
- Attempt to maintain or restore life using CPR when required
- Provide comfort and reassurance to injured athletes
- Activate an emergency plan that includes transfer of treatment responsibility to trained medical personnel
- Complete an injury-report form as soon as possible after an injury occurs

The nine major duties discussed above will help you manage the risk of injury to your athletes and the risk of legal liability to yourself. Two additional recommendations also warrant your consideration.

### Keep Adequate Records

In the event of litigation, it will be essential to have written records to demonstrate that you carried out your legal duties. Practice plans and a record of exactly what was done following an injury, who was notified, and so on, can be critically important.

### Obtain Liability Insurance

As lawsuits have multiplied, the necessity of having adequate liability insurance (at least $1 million worth) has become increasingly evident. Find out what kinds of coverage are provided by your sport program, which should have a policy. If its coverage is inadequate, a low-cost addition to your homeowner's insurance may provide the protection you need.

Obviously, we have merely scratched the surface of sport law in this summary of coaches' legal duties. See the bibliography at the end of the book for several useful sources of additional information.

## COACHING YOUR OWN CHILD

Many volunteer coaches find their way into youth sport programs because their own son or daughter is participating. Therefore, the majority of coaches end up coaching their own child at one time or another. This often results in confusion as to how to deal with the dual roles of coach and parent.

Experienced coaches who have faced this challenge have found a number of principles to be useful. First of all, you and your child need to be aware that your behavior when you are coaching will have to be different than how you behave at home. You now have a responsibility to not only your own child but to all of the other young athletes as well. Recognizing this fact, here are some principles you can follow:

- Ask your child how he or she feels about having you for a coach. Does the child fear undue pressure in the form of either perceived favoritism or excessive demands? If so, give reassurance that you will be fair and impartial and that no more or less will be expected of him or her. Knowing how your child feels will help guide your decision concerning whether your child should be on your team.
- Discuss with your child how your role will change when you are in the athletic environment, and why you need to treat him or her like any other team member.
- Be a parent at home and a coach on the field or court. Make sure that your separate roles are clear in your mind and in your child's mind.
- Above all, demonstrate in your words and actions that your love for your child does not depend on his or her athletic performance.

## COACHING AND FAMILY LIFE

As you are well aware, coaching is very time consuming and takes a lot of energy. Many families find that practices are held during the dinner hour and that their kitchen has become a cafeteria with several shifts. The fun and togetherness of family meals can become a thing of the past. For most families, this is only a seasonal happening. But for coaches who have year-round involvements, it becomes the normal pattern of living. Spouses and children can begin to feel neglected.

When you agree to coach, be aware of what is likely to be required and how much time and effort you are willing to devote. Once into a program, you should also keep in mind that you can easily be seduced into more and more involvement. Before you know it, coaching responsibilities can snowball into a second career, with too little time remaining for your family responsibilities.

Find ways to spend adequate time with your children, particularly those who are not involved in sports. Likewise, it is important for spouses to devote time to their own relationship. For couples who have children, private moments spent away from the children can serve to maintain and invigorate their marriage. Recreational pursuits for you and your spouse, an occasional weekend away by yourselves, dinners out, and a cultivation of interests you share in common can help maintain the sparkle in your marriage.

# Final Words

In chapters 9, 10, and 11, we focused on some of the challenges and negatives of coaching. However, as we ourselves have learned through our coaching experiences, the positives greatly outweigh the negatives. Every problem athlete, problem parent, and coaching headache is outweighed by the moments of satisfaction that come from helping young athletes grow socially, athletically, and personally. Our own children's lives have been enriched by their youth sport experiences.

Although most coaches do not get the credit they rightfully deserve, we know very well that they do indeed make important contributions to the lives of children. And so, our final words are:

Thanks for all you do, and best wishes for a great season!

# Bibliography

## GENERAL RESOURCES

Borkowski, R. P. (1998). *The school sports safety handbook.* Horsham, PA: LRP Publications.

Luiselli, J. K., & Reed, D. D. (Eds.). (2011). *Behavioral sport psychology: Evidence-based approaches to performance enhancement.* New York: Springer.

Martens, R. (2004). *Successful coaching* (3rd ed.). Champaign, IL: Human Kinetics.

Munsey, C. (2010, April). Coaching the coaches: Promoting a "mastery climate" motivates young athletes to do their best, says this scientist-practitioner team. *Monitor on Psychology, 41,* 58–61.

National Council of Youth Sports. (2008). *Report on trends and participation in organized youth sports.* Retrieved from http://www.ncys.org/publications/2008-sports-participation-study.php

National Federation of State High School Associations. (2011). *2010–11 High school athletics participation survey.* Retrieved from http://www.nfhs.org/

Roberts, G. C., Treasure, D. C., & Conroy, D. E. (2007). Understanding the dynamics of motivation in sport and physical activity: An achievement goal interpretation. In G. Tenenbaum & R. C. Eklund (Eds.), *Handbook of sport psychology* (3rd ed., pp. 3–30). New York: Wiley.

Sawyer, T. H. (2001). Legal issues in coaching. In V. Seefeldt & M. A. Clark (Eds.), *Program for athletic coaches' education* (3rd ed., pp. 298–310). Traverse City, MI: Cooper.

Smith, R. E. (2010). A positive approach to coaching effectiveness and performance enhancement. In J. M. Williams (Ed.), *Applied sport psychology: Personal growth to peak performance* (6th ed., pp. 42–58). Boston: McGraw-Hill.

Smith, R. E., & Smoll, F. L. (2005). Assessing psychosocial outcomes in coach training programs. In D. Hackfort, J. L. Duda, & R. Lidor (Eds.), *Handbook of research in applied sport psychology: International perspective* (pp. 293–316). Morgantown, WV: Fitness Information Technology.

Smith, R. E., & Smoll, F. L. (2007). Social-cognitive approach to coaching behaviors. In S. Jowett & D. Lavallee (Eds.), *Social psychology in sport* (pp. 75–90). Champaign, IL: Human Kinetics.

Smith, R. E., & Smoll, F. L. (2011). Cognitive-behavioral coach training: A translational approach to theory, research, and intervention. In J. K. Luiselli & D. D. Reed (Eds.), *Behavioral sport psychology: Evidence-based approaches to performance enhancement* (pp. 227–248). New York: Springer.

Smith, R. E., Smoll, F. L., & O'Rourke, D. J. (2011). Anxiety management. In T. Morris & P. Terry (Eds.), *The new sport and exercise psychology companion* (pp. 227–255). Morgantown, WV: Fitness Information Technology.

Smith, R. E., Smoll, F. L., & Passer, M. W. (2002). Sport performance anxiety in young athletes. In F. L. Smoll & R. E. Smith (Eds.). *Children and youth in sport: A biopsychosocial perspective* (2nd ed., pp. 501–536). Dubuque, IA: Kendall/Hunt.

Smoll, F. L., Cumming, S. P., & Smith, R. E. (2011). Enhancing coach-parent relationships in youth sports: Increasing harmony and minimizing hassle. *International Journal of Sports Science & Coaching, 6,* 13–26.

Smoll, F. L., & Smith, R. E. (Eds.). (2002). *Children and youth in sport: A biopsychosocial perspective* (2nd ed.). Dubuque, IA: Kendall/Hunt.

Smoll, F. L., & Smith, R. E. (2006). Enhancing coach-athlete relationships: Cognitive-behavioral principles and procedures. In J. Dosil (Ed.), *The sport psychologist's handbook: A guide for sport-specific performance enhancement* (pp. 19–37). Chichester, United Kingdom: Wiley.

Smoll, F. L., & Smith, R. E. (2009a). *Mastery approach to coaching: A leadership guide for youth sports.* Seattle, WA: Youth Enrichment in Sports.

Smoll, F. L., & Smith, R. E. (Producers). (2009b). Mastery approach to coaching: A self-instruction program for youth sport coaches [DVD]. Seattle, WA: Youth Enrichment in Sports. http://www.y-e-sports.com

Smoll, F. L., & Smith, R. E. (Producers). (2009c). Mastery approach to parenting in sports: A self-instruction program for youth sport parents [DVD]. Seattle, WA: Youth Enrichment in Sports. http://www.y-e-sports.com

Smoll, F. L., & Smith, R. E. (2010). Conducting psychologically oriented coach-training programs: A social-cognitive approach. In J. M. Williams (Ed.), *Applied sport psychology: Personal growth to peak performance* (6th ed., pp. 392–416). Boston: McGraw-Hill.

*Sports injury risk management: The keys to safety* (2nd ed.). (1998). North Palm Beach, FL: Coalition of Americans to Protect Sports.

Van Raalte, J. L., & Brewer, B. W. (2012). *Exploring sport and exercise psychology* (3rd ed.). Washington, DC: American Psychological Association.

Williams, J. M. (Ed.). (2010). *Applied sport psychology: Personal growth to peak performance* (6th ed.). Boston: McGraw-Hill.

## RESEARCH ARTICLES RELATED TO THE *MASTERY APPROACH TO COACHING*

Barnett, N. P., Smoll, F. L., & Smith, R. E. (1992). Effects of enhancing coach-athlete relationships on youth sport attrition. *The Sport Psychologist, 6,* 111–127.

Cumming, S. P., Smoll, F. L., Smith, R. E., & Grossbard, J. R. (2007). Is winning everything? The relative contributions of motivational climate and won-lost percentage in youth sports. *Journal of Applied Sport Psychology, 19,* 322–336.

Curtis, B., Smith, R. E., & Smoll, F. L. (1979). Scrutinizing the skipper: A study of leadership behaviors in the dugout. *Journal of Applied Psychology*, *64*, 391–400.

Smith, R. E., Shoda, Y., Cumming, S. P., & Smoll, F. L. (2009). Behavioral signatures at the ballpark: Intraindividual consistency of adults' situation-behavior patterns and their interpersonal consequences. *Journal of Research in Personality*, *43*, 187–195.

Smith, R. E., & Smoll, F. L. (1990). Self-esteem and children's reactions to youth sport coaching behaviors: A field study of self-enhancement processes. *Developmental Psychology*, *26*, 987–993.

Smith, R. E., Smoll, F. L., & Barnett, N. P. (1995). Reduction of children's sport performance anxiety through social support and stress-reduction training for coaches. *Journal of Applied Developmental Psychology*, *16*, 125–142.

Smith, R. E., Smoll, F. L., & Cumming, S. P. (2007). Effects of a motivational climate intervention for coaches on children's sport performance anxiety. *Journal of Sport & Exercise Psychology*, *29*, 39–59.

Smith, R. E., Smoll, F. L., & Cumming, S. P. (2009). Motivational climate and changes in young athletes' achievement goal orientations. *Motivation and Emotion*, *33*, 173–183.

Smith, R. E., Smoll, F. L., & Curtis, B. (1978). Coaching behaviors in Little League Baseball. In F. L. Smoll & R. E. Smith (Eds.), *Psychological perspectives in youth sports* (pp. 173–201). Washington, DC: Hemisphere.

Smith, R. E., Smoll, F. L., & Curtis, B. (1979). Coach effectiveness training: A cognitive-behavioral approach to enhancing relationship skills in youth sport coaches. *Journal of Sport Psychology*, *1*, 59–75.

Smith, R. E., Smoll, F. L., & Hunt, E. B. (1977). A system for the behavioral assessment of athletic coaches. *Research Quarterly*, *48*, 401–407.

Smith, R. E., Zane, N. W. S., Smoll, F. L., & Coppel, D. B. (1983). Behavioral assessment in youth sports: Coaching behaviors and children's attitudes. *Medicine and Science in Sports and Exercise*, *15*, 208–214.

Smoll, F. L., & Smith, R. E. (1989). Leadership behaviors in sport: A conceptual model and research paradigm. *Journal of Applied Social Psychology, 19*, 1522–1551.

Smoll, F. L., Smith, R. E., Barnett, N. P., & Everett, J. J. (1993). Enhancement of children's self-esteem through social support training for youth sport coaches. *Journal of Applied Psychology, 78*, 602–610.

Smoll, F. L., Smith, R. E., & Cumming, S. P. (2007a). Effects of a psychoeducational intervention for coaches on changes in child athletes' achievement goal orientations. *Journal of Clinical Sport Psychology, 1*, 23–46.

Smoll, F. L., Smith, R. E., & Cumming, S. P. (2007b, Summer). Effects of coach and parent training on performance anxiety in young athletes: A systemic approach. *Journal of Youth Development, 2*, Article 0701FA002. http://www.nae4ha.org/directory/jyd/index.html

Smoll, F. L., Smith, R. E., Curtis, B., & Hunt, E. (1978). Toward a mediational model of coach-player relationships. *Research Quarterly, 49*, 528–541.

Sousa, C., Smith, R. E., & Cruz, J. (2008). An individualized behavioral goal-setting program for coaches: Impact on observed, athlete-perceived, and coach-perceived behaviors. *Journal of Clinical Sport Psychology, 2*, 258–277.

# Index

# About the Authors

**Ronald E. Smith** is professor of psychology and director of the Clinical Psychology Training Program at the University of Washington. He has also served as head of the Social Psychology and Personality area, and as codirector of the sport psychology graduate program. Professor Smith's major research interests are in personality, stress and coping, and performance enhancement research and intervention. He has published more than 200 scientific articles and book chapters, and he has authored or coauthored 34 books and manuals. Dr. Smith is a fellow of the American Psychological Association, a past president of the Association for Applied Sport Psychology, and the recipient of a Distinguished Alumnus Award from the UCLA Neuropsychiatric Institute for his contributions to the field of mental health. For 12 years, he directed a psychological skills training program for the Houston Astros and has served as Team Counselor for the Seattle Mariners and as a training consultant to the Oakland Athletics and to Major League Soccer.

**Frank L. Smoll** is professor of psychology at the University of Washington and codirector of the sport psychology graduate program. Dr. Smoll's research focuses on coaching behaviors in youth sports and on the psychological effects of competition on children and adolescents. He has authored more than 130 scientific articles and book chapters, and he has coauthored/coedited 22 books and manuals on children's athletics. Professor Smoll is a fellow of the American Psychological Association, the National Academy of Kinesiology, and the Association for Applied Sport Psychology (AASP). Dr. Smoll is an AASP Certified Consultant and was the recipient of AASP's Distinguished Professional Practice Award. As an undergraduate, he played on championship basketball and baseball teams, and he is a member of the Ripon College Athletic Hall of Fame. In the area of applied sport psychology, Dr. Smoll has extensive experience in conducting psychologically oriented coaching clinics and workshops for parents of young athletes.